Dear Carol

Thanks for caring About our

health care system!

Jerry

HEALTH CARE REFORM:

THE TRUTH

HEALTH CARE REFORM:

THE TRUTH

JULIO GONZALEZ, M.D.

Aragon Publishers, Inc.

Venice, Florida

Printed in the United States of America.

Library of Congress Cataloging-in-Publication Data

Gonzalez, Julio, 1964-
       Health Care Reform: The Truth/ Julio Gonzalez. -- 1st ed
           p. ; cm.
       ISBN 978-0-615-26746-3
       1. Health Care Reform   2. Policy

Published and distributed by

Aragon Publishers, Inc.
241 Nokomis Avenue S.
Venice, FL 34285

Additional copies of *"Health Care Reform: The Truth"* (1st ed.) are available from the publisher by sending $29.95 per copy, plus shipping and handling ($8 1st book, $1 each addl.) plus Florida sales tax, if applicable.

*To   America's   Patients,
Present and Future*

Contents

ACKNOWLEDGEMENTS

There are times when events conspire to create opportunities serving to remind us of the smallness of our existence and of the quiet yet all-pervasive presence of the Creator in our world. The events that led to the writing of this book have certainly earned their place in this category. I must therefore start by thanking God for the inspiration, fortitude and discipline necessary to etch these words upon these pages.

No deeper expression of thanks can be extended than to my wife, Dr. Gina Arabitg. There were countless times throughout the writing of this book where doubt and frustration set in only to be dispelled by her strong words of encouragement. It was Gina who would remind me of the need for a platform for the thoughts shared by so many of our colleagues and patients. I have never known her to stand clear while I slaved over a project or manuscript, but this time she did. I once made note of this to her, to which she quickly responded, "Oh, that's because medicine depends on it," reminding me of the great significance of this work to those who agonize over the wellbeing of others.

I must also thank my two daughters, Monica and Jessica, who patiently waited while daddy put everything aside to write this book. And yes, now that I am done with my book, I *will* play basketball with you, Monica, and I *will* help you with that math question, Jessica. Thank you, girls. Everything mom and dad do, they do for *you*!

Among so many other things I learned while writing this book was the meaning of impossible. Impossible means going through this endeavor without the patient and steady support of Ms. Candia Mausser. Candy has been a counselor, proofreader, listener, marketer, layout designer, photo editor, graphics designer, publisher, manager, and everything else. There would be no truth about health care reform without Candy. The story behind her availability to this project is certainly the product of divine manipulation, and I am certainly grateful for that.

I also owe a great deal of gratitude to my good friend and colleague, Dr. Mike Patete. His work in support of medical advocacy has been furious and tireless over the past year, and his example to the rest of us has been monumental. I am deeply indebted to his kind encouragement throughout the development of this book. Not once did he say, "But...", but slowed down long enough to demand that I "get the word out there."

When I called David Lovett, Director of Governmental Affairs at the American Academy of Orthopaedic Surgeons, to solicit his help in this latest of my ideas, he immediately placed all of his resources at my disposal and provided me insight into many of the people behind the politics. I was truly fortunate to have him as a resource, just as medicine is lucky to have him as a friend.

Thanks are also due to Mrs. Linda Cobbe, who reviewed the manuscript at a moment's notice despite it being Christmas and despite all of her other commitments. How she identified that error in the original manuscript is still a mystery to me, but she saved me a great deal of embarrassment in so doing. Someday, she'll tell me how she picked that one up. Her actions certainly serve as testament to her unparalleled attention to detail.

A project of this nature cannot be undertaken without the benefit of having already been deeply immersed in the topic. The door to the arena of health care advocacy was opened to me in 2003 by Fraser Cobbe, Executive Director of the Florida Orthopaedic Society, when he pushed for me to serve as Delegate to the Florida Medical Association. Fraser must have known that I'd be hooked because I haven't looked back since.

Special thanks go to my colleagues at the Florida Orthopaedic Society who have educated me on the ongoing and organized assault on the integrity of our profession, and who have bestowed upon me the privilege of representing them at the state and national levels. I also sincerely thank my fellow Delegates to the Florida Medical Association. Those few days we spend together each year hashing out plans for the future of the House of Medicine are amongst the most educational and insightful of my career.

Thanks mom and dad! It would have never started without you!

Although there are many to thank, there is no one else to blame. The thoughts and ideas expressed in this manuscript are purely my own. I can tell you that they are shared by many of my colleagues, but in the end, I relied on no one to generate these thoughts and recommendations. If there is a flaw in the manuscript or an error in logic or fact, the mistake falls squarely on my shoulders. I can only hope that this effort, however imperfect, will lead the reader to consider alternative viewpoints regarding health care reform to the ones espoused by the so-called reformers of health care, and that it serves as a reminder that the majority of this country's health care providers, the people that spend their lives benefiting from the strengths of our health care system and struggling with its weaknesses, *really* do not want to proceed down the path these reformers are charting.

INTRODUCTION

The 2009 legislative session is sure to be a battlefront for competing interests looking to shape the future of our health care system. The growing concern by the general public and politicians about the increasing costs of health care and of the disparities in its delivery have conspired to make this one of the top priorities for Congress and the incoming administration. Evidence for this is clearly present in the prominent role the issues of health care quality and accessibility played in the 2008 presidential campaigns. The political reality is that those espousing a role for increasing government regulation have, for the first time, entrenched themselves solidly in a position to effect the changes they uphold. The room for effective opposition to this agenda is limited, placing the integrity of the America's health care system more at the mercy of this politically and professionally unidimentional group than ever before.

People who oppose this particular plan for reforming our system share the concerns over health care delivery in this country. They stand resolutely united in the quest to provide better health care in a more efficient and affordable way. However, this group believes that greater government intervention in such a complex and intricate segment of our society will only serve to increase the costs of delivering care and diminish its quality. They hold a view that promotes a stronger role for personal responsibility and accountability in both the delivery and acquisition of health care. They are innately concerned about the future of the American health care workforce and the effects that greater administrative demands and diminished reimbursements will have on the people that deliver this care.

Unfortunately, there is an ocean of misinformation and miscategorization working against this movement. The misrepresentation of the shortcomings of our present health care system is being afforded greater validity by the American public, and attempts at correcting these errors are quickly fading.

Amazingly, the advocates of this alternative viewpoint, the keepers of the more accurate assessment regarding the state of the delivery of our health care, have been egregiously quiet. They will discuss their disappointment over the changes being imparted upon them and their trade in professional conventions and physicians' cafeterias throughout the country. But, either because of despair or simply as a result of a lack of time, these overworked professionals are not voicing their concerns to the public in an effective way. During their meetings, you may hear them warn of the untoward effects government-mandated health care is sure to have on patients and the dissatisfaction with which our citizenry will respond to them. You may even hear these pillars of the health care delivery system discuss their intentions to abandon their careers, or at the very least find a cushion that will allow them to rely less on health care for their livelihood. However, as these individuals dispel from their forums to continue their relentless efforts at caring for others and stem the course of human disease, the microphone is left open for those who have the time such as lawyers, public health experts, economists, academicians and certain legislators, to propagate their brand of misinformation regarding health care in the United States, the overwhelming majority of this group not ever having earned the privilege of laying a stethoscope on a patient.

This book is written in an attempt to reverse the trend of sociopolitical silence on the part of the medical community and as a megaphone for those whose views about health care reform are otherwise not being delivered.

CHAPTER 1:

THE PROBLEM

With increasing vigor, Americans have been debating ways of improving health care delivery in the United States. Advocates for a "repair" or a "fix" of our health care system cite extensive deficiencies in access to care, affordability, and in the quality of health care delivered. Due to a compendium of political circumstances, those who are most convinced of the magnitude of these perceived problems have attained a position where they can effect significant change in the country's health care system with little room for resistance or modification. It is therefore imperative for the American public to study these proposed changes and become intimately aware of their implications so that they may better voice their approval or skepticism of the plans being formulated for them. The effort begins with a review of the problems inherent to our health care delivery system as perceived by the advocates for health care reform.

The United States is presently spending 2.3 trillion dollars on health care, more than 16 percent of its gross domestic product (GDP). The strain this places on the American economy is enormous. Even worse, economists predict that by 2020, this figure will swell to 4 trillion dollars. These exorbitant costs serve to drive up insurance premiums, not only making medical insurance unaffordable to many, but also impeding their ability to pay for their own health care should the need arise.

Julio Gonzalez, M.D.

The mandate of contending with unfunded care adds to this challenge. As of the latest census figures, 15.3 percent of this country's population was uninsured, accounting for 45.7 million people.[1] This rate has decreased slightly compared to 2006 data, but is still unacceptably large. The ethically sound sense of benevolence that drives us to care for our fellow man at great sacrifice to ourselves places a significant financial burden on the health care provider who is legally bound to attend to his uncompensated brethren.[*] In an attempt to ameliorate this daunting financial burden, higher prices are imposed on third-party payers and better funded individuals essentially imposing a hidden tax on these parties.

The problem of insurance undercoverage within our population is not evenly distributed among ethnic and socioeconomic strata. The absence of medical insurance tends to gravitate towards minorities, the poor and children. Whereas Census Bureau data indicated that only 10.8 percent of non-Hispanic whites are uninsured, 19.5 percent of blacks and 32 percent of Hispanics carry a similar burden.[2] It would therefore seem that minority groups, particularly the Hispanic population, are preferentially at risk of being uninsured.

Poverty also served as a negative predictor of an uninsured state. Approximately 25.5% of people living in households earning $25,000 or less are uninsured This compares to 21 percent for individuals living in

* The American Medical Association estimates that the bad debt absorbed per physician from emergency room care is $12,300.00 per year and $138,000.00 per year for each emergency room physician. Source: C.K. Kane, *Physician Marketplace Report: The Impact of EMTALA on Physician Practices* (Chicago: Center for Health Policy Research, American Medical Association, 2003).

households earning $25,000-$49,999; 14.5 percent for individuals living in households earning $50,000-$74,999; and 7.8 percent for individuals living in households earning $75,000 or more.[3] Another group afflicted by uninsurance is children, with an uninsurance rate of 11.0 percent amongst all children and an uninsurance rate of 17.6 percent amongst children living in poverty.[2]

Deficiencies in health care coverage are also associated with poorer levels of care. This relative lack of health care participation leads to fewer preventive medicine measures and a propensity for developing greater severities of disease. The overall effect of these deficiencies is to allow affected individuals to get sicker before seeking care which in turn results in greater amounts of money being spent on their ailments. The financial consequences of such disparities do not remain confined to these groups, however. The increase in overall costs of treatment for these statistically sicker populations places greater strain on the economy and the remaining socioeconomic groups.

The challenge facing lawmakers and policymakers alike is to devise a way of providing health care to our citizenry while maintaining total costs at levels that are affordable to our population and acceptable to taxpayers. Additionally, and concurrent to the main task is the goal of minimizing, if not eradicating, the disparities of access to health care between racial, ethnic, and socioeconomic groups.

As we will see, although the American health care system is imperfect, many of the claims and observations made by proponents of health care reform are at best inaccurate, and many of their proposed solutions merely serve to endanger the integrity of a health care delivery system that is, inarguably, the most sophisticated and responsive in the world.

CHAPTER 2:

HOW THE HEALTH CARE SYSTEM PRESENTLY RUNS

Health Care Funding

The United States health care industry is a mixed payer system funded by a combination of private and public entities. In 2007, approximately 202 million people were covered by private health insurance (67.5 percent).[1] Within the private sector, there was a high reliance on employer based insurance coverage with 177.3 million people (59.3 percent) receiving their private insurance through their employer. Eighty-three million people (27.8 percent) were covered by government-sponsored insurance programs, with Medicare covering 41.4 million people (13.8 percent), Medicaid covering 39.6 million people (13.2 percent), and the military health care system covering 10.95 million (3.7 percent).[1]

The Workforce

As of 2005, there were 817,500 practicing physicians in the United States.[4] Of these, 306,100 (37.4 percent) worked in the primary care-related fields (areas such as internal medicine, pediatrics, and family practice). The rest were specialists. In 2000, there were 2,201,800 registered nurses, amounting to 807.4 nurses per 100,000 people.[5] Additionally, there were countless other ancillary service providers ranging from dieticians to medical environmental-service workers.

Physicians represent an indispensable commodity for the country, encompassing the most sophisticated, highly-educated, and skilled elements of our society. Each physician represents the product of a minimum of 23 years of training. This includes 12 years of standard schooling (grade school through high school), four years of college education, four years of medical school training and, on the average, a minimum of 3 years of postgraduate education (residency training).

Physicians who pursue specialty training usually trade those three years of residency for five to eight years of postgraduate training in their selected specialty. A general practice physician is about 29 years of age when he completes his training. Specialty physicians are between 31 and 35 years of age by the time their training is complete. As a result of their efforts, physicians amass between $120,588.00 and $265,472.00 purely on education-based debt.[6,7] This, of course, does not include lost earnings during the years spent in training and vastly underestimates the amount that society invests in producing the physician.

As health care cannot be delivered without the services of these dynamic professionals, they represent the central link of any health care system model. One can redesign the reimbursement schemes, or the hospitals, or even the insurance networks, but in the end, care cannot be delivered without the presence and participation of a vibrant physician workforce.

Equally, physicians cannot deliver care without the assistance of nurses. These too are highly motivated, intelligent, exceedingly altruistic individuals with an ingrained devotion to service. They undergo four years of post-high school training before entering the workforce. They are generally employed as salaried workers and usually are not in positions where they are taking the financial risks of running their own free-standing businesses as do many American physicians. They generally finish their studies in their early twenties and as such, have a longer productive lifespan than do physicians. Like physicians, the training attained by these individuals is intense, and many go on to achieve subspecialty training at the expense of more time and money. Such specialty interests include operating room nurses, obstetrical nurses, triage nurses, nurse anesthetists, and independent nurse practitioners to name a few.

Like many other segments of our society, physicians

and nurses are in short supply, particularly those in certain key specialties and geographical regions.[8] To make matters worse, the country's aging pattern stands to worsen the disparity between the number of health care professionals and the general population. By the year 2020, the number of people living in the United States who are above 65 years of age is expected to increase by 50 percent, while the physician population is expected to grow by a meager 16 percent. [4] Compounding the problem is the concurrent aging pattern of the physician population. One study performed in Florida in 2007 found the average age of physicians practicing in that state to be 51.43 years with many specialties having older mean ages.[9]. As a result, any changes in the health care system must provide sufficient incentives for these individuals to remain in practice as a massive exodus of the older ranks of practicing physicians would not be tolerated by the health care delivery system.

Our medical schools are cognizant of the increasing workloads America's aging population will bring and have stepped up their efforts at increasing the volume of physicians produced each year. The numbers of medical students graduating from American schools each year has increased by 11.58 percent from 1997 to 2008.[10] Additionally, the total number of enrollments in American medical schools has risen by 6.67 percent between 2002 and 2005, to 70,225 students.

The United States has also increased its reliance on foreign medical graduates (FMGs).[11] Since 1978, the number of FMGs in our workforce has grown by 4,873 physicians per year to a total of 215,576 in 2004, or 25.6 percent of the actively practicing physician population.

As a whole this group is less likely to be board-certified, more likely to practice internal medicine and work in underserved areas than American-trained physicians. The leading source countries from which the United States imports its foreign medical graduates are India, the Philippines, and Mexico.[12] Although significant differences exist between foreign and American-trained physicians studies have not conclusively determined any significant differences in the quality of care delivered by FMGs when compared to their American-trained counterparts.[13s]

Julio Gonzalez, M.D.

*How Physicians Get Paid**

Physician reimbursement is a complex and mysterious process, even to physicians. Essentially, physicians bill insurance companies through codes of services, known as "current procedural terminology codes" or CPT codes. These codes help to standardize the different services provided by physicians into a common communication modality. Essentially, everything that a physician does, from seeing a patient in the office all the way to the most complex surgery is given a CPT code number. Additionally, there are CPT codes that allow physicians to bill nonsurgical interactions with patients, known as "evaluation and management" (E&M) codes. Most E&M codes carry a one-day global period of service, meaning that the service provided covers all actions performed by that physician for that day. Many procedural codes, particularly the surgery codes, carry a 90-day global period, meaning that payment for that procedure includes compensation for 90-days worth of routine following-up.

* For the sake of brevity, physician reimbursement methods are discussed here. Similar methods are in place for different health care providers. Reimbursement procedures are roughly similar for institutions such as hospitals and nursing homes with each carrying their particular nuances specific to their roles in providing care.

When a physician performs a service, the CPT code that best describes that service is submitted to the third party payer (insurance company) along with a corresponding diagnosis code. Take, for example, a patient who presents to the office of a physician he has never met before for treatment of a cold. The physician evaluates the patient, comes up with a treatment plan and provides the patient with the appropriate treatment. The physician then bills for an initial outpatient evaluation and treatment session using the appropriate E&M CPT code (either a 99203 or a 99204 depending on the level of the complexity of the evaluation). The physician would also need to inform the insurance company of the diagnosis that he treated, so along with the CPT code, a diagnosis code, or ICD code (International Classification of Diseases code), would also be provided[†]. Those charges may be communicated to the third party payer either electronically or by mail depending on the resources available to either party.

Once those charges are submitted, the insurance company typically takes about two to six weeks to review it, approve it, and send out the payment. Of course, the insurance company can just as easily ask for more documentation, such as the office notes, in order to validate the claim. There is also no guarantee that the insurance company will pay the claim, asserting that the service rendered was not a covered service. As a matter of fact, even if the payer authorized the treatment prior to it being delivered, and even if physician and patient are able to provide an authorization number to validate the claim, the third-party payer still generally reserves

[†] Presently, the working codes through which the medical industry commu-
nicates are in their ninth revision thus earning them the name ICD9 codes

the right to reject the claim. Although this infrequently happens, it is a particularly strong point of contention for patient and provider alike.

The amount paid to the physician is usually agreed upon by the physician and the third party payer ahead of time by contractual agreement. This amount usually is not the amount the physician regularly charges for a service and is listed in a "fee schedule". This "schedule" is a list of compensations the payer is agreeing to pay the physician for each and every CPT code billed. This is done first by assigning each CPT code a "relative value unit" or RVU. This is an estimation of the amount of work and risk to the provider required to perform a certain procedure. One can assign whatever RVU one likes to any procedure, but the insurance industry generally uses the RVU scheme used by the Centers for Medicare and Medicaid Services (CMS)[‡]. CMS relies on the American Medical Association's Relative Value Unit Committee to devise its RVU list and updates it every five years. The RVU for each CPT code is then multiplied by a conversion factor that gives the payer, patient and provider a final reimbursement fee for each procedure or interaction. The final fee schedule generally runs about 30 percent to 50 percent of the physician's usual and customary charges, thus providing the patient and the payer a sizeable discount for the physician's services in exchange for the provider's privilege of accessing those patients.

Other payment formulas exist that dictate physician reimbursement. One of the more popular is the "per

[‡]   The Centers for Medicare and Medicaid Services (CMS) is that agency of the federal government created as part of the Social Security Act of 1965 to manage the Medicare and Medicaid insurances.

capita" model, where the third party payer pays the physician for the number of enrollees in the insurance plan. The physician gets paid the same amount regardless of whether he sees those patients or not and regardless of the amount of work he performs on those patients. Capitated plan formulas strive to induce the physician into cutting down on the number of unnecessary or frivolous tests and services provided.

A few interesting side notes are worthy of mention regarding physician reimbursement. The first relates to the power that CMS has in controlling the amount that physicians get paid. It is CMS that devises and approves the different coding plans. As such, CMS defines the services provided by physicians and assigns them relative values. The insurance industry looks to CMS as a reference on the relative values of the different procedures as well as to the actual amount paid. In fact, many companies negotiate physician reimbursement fee schedules as a percentage of Medicare payments, thus establishing CMS and the federal government as the benchmark for reimbursement methods and levels of provider reimbursement.

The other interesting peculiarity relates to the federal antitrust legislation. Under federal law, it is illegal for two physicians in the same market to discuss reimbursement rates unless they belong to the same group or business. Insurance companies, however, are allowed to discuss reimbursement rates with each other, including information regarding the different reimbursement rates acceptable to each physician. This dicotomy in how the law treats the different parties of the health care industry results in a distinct disadvantage to the provider and severely inhibits his ability to negotiate on even terms with the corporate giants that inherently hold the fiscal advantage on the market.

Accessing Care

Access to health care in the United States is fairly straightforward, and the response time is better than that of any other country in the world.[14] Americans tend to wait less time than in any other developed country for elective procedures.[14,15] Even the World Health Organization, which is very quick to aim their criticisms at the American health care system, rates the United States as having *the* most responsive health care system in the world.[14] The percentage of people waiting more than four months for non-emergency surgery in the United States is about one tenth that of the nearest contender.[16] Additionally, the percentage of patients receiving elective surgery with less than one month of wait time is the highest in the word.[16] Such ease of accessibility is arguably the strongest advantage of the American health care system.

The patient needing emergency service can seek care, through the approximately 3,833 emergency departments in this country. As will be discussed later in this book, access to these centers is guaranteed regardless of one's ability to pay.[15]

The ability to achieve responsiveness of this kind obviously costs money and may serve as the single most important explanation for the high cost of health care in this country, as a tight correlation exists between a health care system's responsiveness and a country's per capita health care expenditure.[17]

The Scope of the Uninsured

The fact that there are 46 million uninsured people living in the United States is often used to discredit the American health care system. It is felt that any society allowing 13.7 percent of its population to go without access to health care is not truly advanced. However, many within this group are ones who can afford health care coverage but simply choose not to purchase it. Appropriately, most taxpayers would not feel responsible for paying for the health care coverage of this affluent segment of society. Therefore, a more appropriate question is for which individuals living in the United States should the government and taxpayer be assisting with the procurement of health care coverage. An attempt at answering this question will reveal vastly different numbers than the ones many advocates of sweeping health care reform would prefer that we believe.

First, 38.6 percent of uninsured individuals living in the United States, or 17,603,000 people, reside in households earning more than $50,000.00 per year.[3] Another 29.7 percent, or 13,539,000 individuals, are living below the federal poverty level. A large number of these are eligible for Medicaid services. This leaves 32.8 percent of uninsured individuals, or 14,515, 000 people living in households that earn between $25,000.00 and $49,999,99. Members of these last two groups are at significant risk of not being able to pay their medical bills should they get sick, and not being able to afford health care insurance despite their desire to procure it.[3]

Adding to the uncertainty of the problem is the inaccuracy of Census data. The American Census cannot differentiate between individuals who are living in the country legitimately and those estimated 11.8 million people who are living in this country illegally.[18] This is an important distinction as most Americans oppose public funding of health care for illegal immigrants.[19] It is safe to assume that the majority of individuals who are residing in this country illegally belong to overtly poor households or to lower middle class families. Although we are not able to ascertain the distribution of these illegal immigrants between the two lowest economic strata, we can say that of the 28.1 million uninsured individuals who reside in either poverty or lower middle class households, only 16.3 million (28.1million total individuals in these two economic groups minus the 11.8 million individuals who are residing in this country illegally) are individuals for whom Americans could foster a politically significant level of support towards the funding of health care coverage. Even this number is inflated as a certain percentage of this group is already eligible for publicly funded health care coverage. Those legitimate advocates for health care reform should not allow the 11.8 million people residing in this country illegally to cloud the picture of the true magnitude of health care uninsurance. Decisions regarding policy toward illegitimate inhabitants require a broader approach, not just one limited to health care coverage and access.

There is a small but important second group of uninsureds in this country for whom there is significant popular support: the "uninsurables". These are individuals who do not have access to government or employer-sponsored insurance plans but are unable to purchase individual health care insurance plans due to the presence of underlying conditions or health risks that are deemed unacceptable to private insurers. Surprisingly, there is no reliable data on the number of "uninsurables" in this country. However, data from the Health Insurance Resource Center indicate that this number is substantial, as 134,000 Americans find themselves in high-risk state pools throughout the 34 states that have them.[20,21] Collectively, these 34 states encompass 59 percent of the country's population.[22] Assuming a similar medically-uninsurable rate throughout all states, (an admittedly scientifically invalid assumption), then the total number of medically-uninsurable individuals can be estimated to run at least 226,460 people. If we presume that between 20 and 50 percent of the medically-uninsurable population participates in the high-risk pool for each state, we can then surmise that the total number of people in this country who are not eligible for either employer-based or government-sponsored insurance programs and are deemed to be medically-uninsurable ranges from 452,480 to 1,132,300 individuals.

Julio Gonzalez, M.D.

The Health Care Guarantee

The health care guarantee results from a pledge made by the government and health care providers to all inhabitants in this country. It is the product of the great sense of benevolence of the American people and the responsibility that they feel towards the well-being of their fellow man and upholds a pillar of respect and honor to the human condition and to the value of human life. It is a manifestation of feelings of community and devotion to one's neighbors that helped forge a civilization out of dense forests and uncharted territory. It is the great equalizer in the charge of an absence of universal health care in this country, and it is one that is backed by the full authority of the federal government[§]. The guarantee essentially holds that no matter who you are, how you found yourself in this country, or what your

§ In 1986, the federal government passed the Consolidated Omnibus Budget Reconciliation Act (COBRA) which includes a section known as the Emergency Medical Treatment and Active Labor Act (EMTALA) upholding that all hospitals had the responsibility to perform an extensive screening examination to any patient presenting with any medical condition regardless of his ability to pay. It specifically stipulates that this screening test has to be more extensive than merely a triage evaluation. Additionally, the hospital was mandated to maintain an on-call system (doctors, nurses, etc) to assist in the stabilization of these patients. It also stipulated that the hospital was responsible to provide the full complement of its resources towards the stabilization of these patients.

ability to pay may be, if you find yourself in a medical situation that you feel is urgent or emergent, you will be cared for in an emergency room by the full resources and expertise available to the institution responsible for that department.

Despite the difficulties that this pledge imparts on the emergency rooms of this country and those covering them, this is a commitment of which we can be supremely proud. It is also one that, as is explained elsewhere in this book, is not shared universally by all societies. From a health policy standpoint, it is one that essentially imposes an imperfect but complete universal access clause to our health care system. It guarantees that all *inhabitants* have access to an essential element of health care, and, as evidenced by the types of unfunded cases that present to our nation's emergency rooms each year, it does not even require that the case be emergent in nature. Health policy students and experts call this "unfunded" care, but whether we wish to acknowledge it or not, the care is actually funded, whether formally or not.

The problem with the mandate is that it is very expensive and inefficient. Dollar for dollar, the emergency room is the most expensive place in which to provide routine care. The resources expended on emergency room care are large compared to those provided by free-standing facilities. Adding to the inefficiency is the fact that personnel and resources employed in addressing non-emergent care tie up access to legitimate emergencies. Individuals presenting to the emergency room for non-urgent medical conditions help to inappropriately drive up the costs of providing care, slow down the progression of legitimate cases through the emergency room and over-task individuals whose energies are best directed at life or limb threatening situations. Unfortunately, however, federal law prohibits emergency rooms from turning even these inappropriate presentations away, so these institutions are forced to treat these cases despite the inefficiencies they may impart upon the health care delivery system.

It is because of this pledge and the federal mandate that backs it up that the deficiency being discussed regarding our health care system does not relate to an absence of universal access or universal care as such access already exists in our country, and through the hidden methods of funding, one can even argue that it has a really inefficient system of "universal coverage". The true discussion about the universality of health care in this country is appropriately centered about the efficiency with which our heath care is delivered, the types of noneconomic resources being employed in providing this care, and its cost.

A few examples will go a long way towards solidifying this point. An illegal immigrant who was being transported to a political rally on illegal immigration fell off the back of a pick-up truck on I-75 while traveling at speeds in excess of 70 miles per hour. The patient sustained complex and life-threatening injuries, including fractures to three of his extremities, each requiring surgical intervention. The injury occurred early in the morning. The orthopaedic surgeon on duty for the emergency room was called to address the situation. The physician, seeing the extent and urgency of the problem canceled his full day of scheduled patients and spent the day attending to the patient...over eight hours of surgery. It was obvious that this patient would not be able to pay for his care. Regardless, the physician had to cancel his office and attend to the patient's injuries, losing thousands of dollars of income and inconveniencing dozens of patients who were scheduled to see the doctor, all over a patient who wasn't even supposed to be in this country and was on his way to protest the immigration policies of the country whose resources he was now about to hoard.

Contrast this with the situation in Somalia. During the Somalian invasion of 1993, the United States military was sent to perform humanitarian operations by providing basic health services to the area's indigent population. I was one of the physicians sent ashore to care for Somali patients . While there, a middle-aged man brought his young wife to us for care. The woman was at death's door, being transported to our compound on a wheel barrel.

We immediately took care of her, providing her intravenous hydration and antibiotics. Over the ensuing two days, the woman regained her strength such that she was able to walk again. We were able to discontinue her IV antibiotics and her intravenous fluids, and switched her to oral medications. Throughout the span of those three days, her husband would visit her daily. During one of those encounters, I asked her husband why it was that he had not taken her to the hospital. He said it was because he had no money noting that without it, the hospital would not let him set foot through their doors. He explained to me that even in the state in which his wife had been, literally hours away from dying, their hospital would have allowed her to die in the front steps of its doors rather than take care of her.

Julio Gonzalez, M.D.

This is truly what is meant by not having access to health care, not what we encounter in our country.

Medicare

On November 19, 1945, as part of his address to Congress, President Harry S. Truman proposed a plan to improve the state of health care in this country. The idea would call for the creation of a national health insurance that would cover all workers. According to his vision, the plan would require no federal moneys and would cost $1.00 per month for each worker with a matched contribution from the employer. A fund would therefore be established that would assist workers in paying their medical bills. The physician, according to President Truman, "would not be interfered with in any way".[23]

Needless to say, the enormity of the vast number of projected beneficiaries and the socialist undertones of the program led to great opposition from many fronts including the American Medical Association and the American Hospital Association. Ultimately, the national health insurance plan did not pass, but remained alive in the halls of Congress to be revised and debated.

In 1965, under the presidency of Lyndon B. Johnson, what started as a national health insurance plan for workers was finally established as a health care plan for seniors through the Social Security Act of 1965. The law established Medicare as an indemnity health insurance plan for Social Security recipients and created the Medicaid system, designed to provide assistance for our nation's poor.

Predictably, Medicare grew in scope. In 1972, Medicare was expanded to include coverage for disabled individuals who were younger than 65.[24] In 1980, home health service coverage was expanded and supplemental insurance coverage was created. In 1982, legislation was passed to facilitate the abilities of health maintenance organizations to contract with Medicare. In 1982, the Catastrophic Coverage Act increased hospital and skilled nursing facility benefits, but was repealed the following year in response to protests from elderly patients because of the higher premiums the plan would require. Over the years, what started as a vision for a supplemental health care fund for workers grew into the largest health care payer in this country covering 13.8 million Americans and carrying an annual budget of $260 billion or 17 percent of U.S. expenditures.[25]

Arguably more important than its impact relating to its sheer size is the role Medicare and the Centers for Medicare and Medicaid Services (the program that manages Medicare) have taken as regulators of our health care industry. In 1989, legislation went into effect that established a new fee schedule for physician reimbursement. The same legislation also prohibited physicians from balance-billing for their services.¶

¶ Balance-billing is the practice of billing the patient for the differences between the reimbursement paid by a third-party payer and the provider's usual and customary charge for that service. Prohibiting balance billing protects the insured from having to pay more for a service than that negotiated (or in the case of Medicare-mandated) by the insurer. It also imparts great power upon the insurer in determining reimbursement rates for the provider.

Additionally, physicians were no longer allowed to refer Medicare patients to clinical laboratories where they had a financial stake, expanding the ever-increasing encroachment of federal regulations into the private sector.

In 1996, the Health Insurance Portability and Accountability Act added provisions regarding portability and privacy regulations that placed restrictions not just on Medicare participants, but on private insurers as well. It also required CMS to enact privacy regulations should Congress fail to enact them itself, furthering the regulatory capacity of this agency.

The 1997 Balanced Budget Act provided CMS with more powers. These included a greater informational and educational role, the creation of five new prospective payment systems for Medicare (for inpatient rehabilitation hospital or unit services, skilled nursing facility services, home health services, hospital outpatient department services, and outpatient rehabilitation services), expanded preventive services, and allowed CMS to test innovative approaches for payment through research and demonstrations.

In 2003, the Medicare Prescription Drug Improvement and Modernization Act provided coverage for prescription drugs, allowing for federal subsidies for employers who provided Medicare-like prescription drug coverage, and for the first time, allowing for the adjustment of Medicare premiums for higher-income seniors.

In this way, the meager, $2.00 per month program that would have no restrictive function on how physicians delivered care and would serve only to pay for physician and hospital services was turned into a mammoth government program of spending, oversight, and market manipulation that is the primary influence on how health care is delivered today.[26]

And there is still much controversy over the benefits of the Medicare system. The late Dr. Douglas Murphy echoes the sentiments of countless physicians regarding the implementation of Medicare in his 1994 article that appeared in the Venice Gondolier.[27] In it, Dr. Murphy prophetically said, "Long before the birth of Medicare, I never saw a patient in need go untreated...The Federal Government unnecessarily decided to pay doctors for surgery they were willing to do *gratis*. We doctors felt that this was not out of goodness of the Federal heart, but rather a deceitful way to begin the destruction of our independence. The divide and conquer game was on its way. The prescription for Big Government in medicine was born."

And there is objective evidence to support this contention. Amy Finkelstein in her reviews on the topic found that the introduction of Medicare resulted in a 23 percent increase in hospital expenditures between 1965 and 1970.[28] She also estimated that Medicare may single-handedly have been responsible for 40 percent of the increased per-capita health care spending that took place in the United States between 1965 and 1990. Additionally, there is doubt over whether the decrease in elderly mortality rates that took place during the first five years after the establishment of the Medicare program had anything to do with Medicare at all. Studies suggest that Medicare had little impact on elderly mortality in the United States during the first ten years of its existence.[29]

The reason for this is that prior to Medicare, as Dr. Murphy reports, elderly patients were seeking medical attention for their conditions so long as they had legal access to hospitals. According to historical experience, the result of government intervention in the health care system may have been to induce the very same effects it was trying to avoid. In other words, government planning, study, regulation and intervention may have caused our system to be more expensive and more difficult to manage than it would have been without it.

It can certainly be said that government intervention has made the plight of the health care provider more difficult. The Balanced Budget Act of 1997 mandated that the Medicare Economic Index (MEI) as adjusted by the Sustainable Growth Rate formula (SGR) be the formula through which physician reimbursement would be determined. The MEI is an index that determines physician input (investment) into health care delivery (essentially the cost of practicing medicine). The Balanced Budget of 1997 called for this figure to be adjusted by the SGR, which is a target rate on health care expenditure based on natural economic indicators such as the GDP. The result would be a figure that would determine the amount of moneys paid to physicians for their services while balancing the costs of practicing medicine with the need to keep medical spending shifts from drifting out of control. The final number, called the updated adjustment factor (UAF), would be used to modify physician reimbursement on a yearly basis and would be due in Congress by March 1st of each year. The equation used to calculate the UAF is listed below with the applicable numbers for 2009.[30]

$$\text{UAF}_{\text{(for the year)}} = \frac{\text{Target}_{\text{(prior year's)}} - \text{Actual}_{\text{(prior year's)}}}{\text{Actual}_{\text{(prior year's)}}} \times 0.75 + \frac{\text{Target}_{\text{(4/96-12/08)}} - \text{Actual}_{\text{(4/96-12/08)}}}{\text{Actual}_{\text{(4/96-12/08)}}} \times 0.33$$

$\text{Target}_{\text{(prior year's)}}$ = Estimated Allowed Expenditures for prior year. ($86.8 billion for 2008).
The target expenditures is the allowed expenditure for the year and is the annual allowed expenditures for the previous year increased by SGR.[105]
$\text{Actual}_{\text{(prior year's)}}$ = Estimated Actual Expenditures for the prior year. ($94.4 billion for 2008).
$\text{Target}_{\text{(4/96-12/08)}}$ = Estimated Cumulative Allowed Expenditures from 4/1/96 - 12/31/08 = $863.7 billion
$\text{Actual}_{\text{(4/96-12/08)}}$ = Estimated Cumulative Actual Expenditures from 4/1/96 - 12/31/08 = $926.8 billion
SGR_{2009} = Estimated Sustainable Growth Rate for 2009 = 7.4 percent or 0.074

The UAF for 2009 is therefore -0.266, or -26.6 percent. However, since there is a mandated cap on the UAF of not greater than 3 percent and not less than 7 percent. The UAF for 2009 therefore will be -7 percent.

The final physician's fee schedule adjustment is determined by aggregating the UAF for the year with the MEI for the year (the MEI for 2009 is 1.6 percent). In the case of 2009, the adjustment to the physician fee schedule is -5.5 percent, and only because the actual calculated UAF of -26.6 percent is not being used, as the rules hold that negative UAF values are to be capped at 7 percent. Otherwise, the answer would have been -25.0 percent.

The SGR has called for a reduction in physician reimbursements every year since 2002. On more than one occasion the reductions have been sizeable resulting in a significant threat to continued physician involvement in the Medicare system and erosion of senior citizens' access to health care. These consistently negative answers to the formula have come at a time when the cost of providing health care has predictably increased. If physician and health care provider reimbursement cuts had been implemented at rates similar to the ones calculated, clinicians would no longer be able to provide care on a financially sustainable basis.

Recognizing this, Congress has mandated delays in the implementation of the calculated cuts almost on a yearly basis. However, with each delay, a cumulative effect is absorbed that includes the budgetary effects of prior mandated delays. As such, under the current guidelines, with the cumulative effects of all prior cuts still in effect, the reimbursement cut for physicians scheduled to take place in January 2010 is 20.1 percent and 41 percent by 2016. It must be noted that despite these periodic congressional adjustments, inflation-corrected physician reimbursement since 1995 has still diminished by 44 percent.[**]

The effect has been to inject uncertainty and instability into the Medicare-dependent health care markets. Physicians have hesitated to migrate to states with high Medicare populations such as Florida. Additionally, practices in these areas have hesitated to recruit new physicians or expand their services. Increasingly, physicians are making accommodations such as planning for early retirement in case the threatened scheduled Medicare reimbursement cuts are implemented.

As noted previously, the effects of Medicare reimbursement ripple throughout the health care market as private payers look at Medicare to guide them in setting their respective fee schedules and policies. In areas of the country where Medicare patients encompass a large percentage of the population, physicians are not in

[**]   It should be noted that this figure is for total reimbursement. The take-home pay cuts for physicians are actually greater once one includes overhead deductions.

a position to negotiate with the private payers because all payers know that these physicians are willing to accept the Medicare-contracted rates for their services. In knowing how much these physicians are accepting from the government they are provided with an advantage against the providers in setting their fees. Physicians in these Medicare intense markets are essentially at the mercy of congressional policy, not just to determine the reimbursement rates for their Medicare patients, but also, to a large degree the fee schedules from the private payers.

From the provider's standpoint, the overall effect of Medicare has been to decrease reimbursement while increasing the regulatory burden and cost of practicing medicine, all to address a perceived problem that many physicians of the time contended not to have existed, or at the very least, did not merit being addressed in the sweeping manner in which it ultimately was. Whereas in other industries and professions, the provider of the service or product is allowed to adjust his rates as dictated by market pressures and risk-assessments, in the medical industry, the reimbursement rates are essentially mandated by the government and large corporations, removing any possibility of the provider adjusting his prices in response to the costs of running his practice. The result has been to make the business of practice medicine unsustainable in many markets, particularly those with an abundant Medicare or indigent population.

Medicaid

The Medicaid system possesses significant differences from Medicare. For one, Medicaid is a social assistance program designed to help those who are living in poverty and/or have special needs. Although Medicare is a strictly federal program, funding for Medicaid is shared by the federal and state governments. Its administration is the responsibility of the state governments under the coordination of CMS and does vary between states. Approximately 13.2 percent of the population's health care is covered by state Medicaid programs. Adults must be American citizens of low income, authorized immigrants, blind or pregnant in order to be eligible. However, living in poverty is not grounds for automatic Medicaid eligibility. Children living in the United States under authorized conditions are eligible to participate in Medicaid regardless of the eligibility status of their parents. Problems with insufficient provider participation largely due to low reimbursement rates and administrative hassles are some of the challenges facing the Medicaid health care delivery system.

The United States Department
of Veterans Affairs

Formerly known as Veterans Administration, the system was established July 21, 1930. The mission of the department is, as stated by Abraham Lincoln, "to care for him who shall have borne the battle, and for his widow and his orphan." The Veterans Health Administration, a subdivision of the Department of Veterans Affairs, essentially represents a single-payer, government-run health care system with a budget of $90 billion. It is the largest integrated health care system in the United States.[31] The levels of care differ depending on income, degree of service and disability. Veterans with greater than a 50 percent service-related disability rating are eligible for comprehensive medical coverage inclusive of prescription medications.

Long delays in access to care have plagued the VA system in the past. These faults, however, may be as much due to insufficient staffing and funding concerns as to any inherent troubles of a universal health care system. Fairly or not, issues regarding inefficiency and poor productivity related to the VA system have been used as examples of the disadvantages of government-run health care schemes.

The Veterans Health Care Eligibility Reform Act of 1996 tasked the system with reforming itself from a hospital system to a health care system. This was accomplished using Veterans Integrated Service Networks (VISNs) transforming the impetus of the health care to the outpatient setting. The care delivered by the Veterans Health Administration is now much more coordinated and centered on preventive measures. It is hoped that with these reforms the Veterans Health Administration will vastly improve the way health care is administered to our veterans.

Julio Gonzalez, M.D.

The Military Health Care System

The military's health care system covers about 3.7 percent of the population, mostly composed of individuals in active duty service, their families, and some retirees. It is an integrated, universally-applied, singly-administered health care system full of mandated interventions such as vaccinations and routine physical examinations. It is also goal oriented. Specifically, it is designed to promote military readiness and minimize casualties due to sickness and disease. Because of the uniqueness of this system and its purposes, its structure and make-up have limited applicability to health care directed at the general population.

Medical Malpractice

Medical malpractice, or the threat thereof, places an immeasurable burden on the American health care system. The crux of the problem lies in medicine's inherent imperfections and in its prospective nature. Civil law, on the other hand, is a retrospective field, one that always questions what could have been done differently and second-guesses the actions of those bold enough to take them. The retrospection, however, is not undertaken with the aim of improving performance as is done in peer review exercises and medical seminars. This exercise is carried out with the sole, unproductive, and shameless purpose of assigning blame and making money.

At the heart of this endemic is a moral milieu that infests our society promoting the justice system not as a bastion of righteousness, but as a conduit for quick money. What's worse, medical malpractice attorneys, who are supposed to be the beacon of fairness and justice, see the constant flow of disappointed patients and disgruntled loved ones as income-generating opportunities, knowing that as long as they have a stream of clients, they stand to make money off the system whether they win a case or not.

As such, advertisements for medical malpractice attorneys and personal injury lawyers pervade our environment, encouraging us to call should we find any reason to be dissatisfied with any medical experience. If we open a telephone book we see them, not just in the attorneys section, but in every corner of each page as well as in the inside and outside back covers. Their faces decorate our cities' billboards adorned with catchy slogans of how they are here to defend *you* against the big guys, including your doctor...who generally isn't very big at all. And most distressingly, they are in the television, blaring in the hospital room, oftentimes serving as background noise to the physician while he is trying to deliver care instructions to the patient.

To these attorneys, the important thing is to keep arguing, for as long as they can do that, there is the possibility of accessing the deep pocket, one that they know is all-too-willing to pay just to make them go away. These lawyers do not serve as "counselors" as they enjoy being called, but enablers, assisting their clients in pursuing their claim, whether the suit carries merit or not.

Providers are well aware of the environment in which they practice and feel compelled to institute protective measures. One such action is to obtain medical malpractice insurance designed to finance one's defense in case of a lawsuit and pay for damages in light of an unfavorable judgment. Like in any other form of insurance, any factor identified by the insurer that places the provider at higher risk of litigation or adverse outcome is translated into an increase in premium. Such factors include prior actions against the physician, number of years in practice[††], specific specialty of practice, and the litigious pattern of the community the physician is serving. The result is that insurance premiums for 250/750 coverage[‡‡] generally run as inexpensively as $15,000 per year for the lower-risk, nonsurgical specialties, to upwards of $100,000 per year for higher-risk specialties such as obstetrics, neurosurgery, orthopaedic surgery, trauma surgery and general surgery. These exorbitant premiums get added on to the provider's overhead, compounding the pressure to see more patients and to see them faster, driving up the cost of health care delivery while diminishing the quality of that care.

And the size of these premiums is on the rise. The Congressional Budget Office noted an overall increase of 15 percent in medical malpractice premiums for physicians nationwide between 2000 and 2002, with certain specialties such as obstetrics, internal medicine, and general surgery being hit harder.[32] The average payment as a result of awards has also risen dramatically from an average of $95,000 in 1986 to $320,000 in 2002, largely accounting for the associated rise in premiums.[33]

It is therefore understandable for physicians to do everything in their power to keep their malpractice risk as low as possible. One way of doing this is by engaging in defensive medicine tactics. This is the practice of ordering more and sometimes unnecessary tests in

[††] Ironically, in the insurance world, being a young, inexperienced physician translates to a lower risk of coverage than for the more senior, physician due to the smaller history of interactions covered.

[‡‡] $250,000.00 of coverage for each event, $750,000.00 of coverage maximum per year.

order to remove as many doubts as possible of alternate diagnoses, or sometimes, merely to make "the chart look good for the attorneys". These actions are a direct result of pressure placed on providers to be prepared to defend themselves in case of a bad outcome.

According to the Congressional Budget Office, however, the effects of defensive medicine are fairly small, basing its conclusions on the findings of the Harvard Medical Practice Study, an outdated report published in 1990 and one whose validity has been questioned.[34] The CBO goes on to conclude that medical malpractice and medical malpractice reform has little effect on health care spending. This position is taken as valid and repeated in "Call to Action."[35]

Another step the provider can take in reducing his malpractice risk is, ironically enough, not to buy malpractice insurance. The option of "self-insuring" or "going bare" is one that is regulated at the state level and therefore varies between states with some states not even permitting the option. By going bare, the physician places himself and his family at great financial risk. However, that risk is offset by his diminished attractiveness as a lawsuit recipient. However, as the percentage of self-insured physicians grows, the legal community has become increasingly aggressive in its pursuit of the self-insured physician, despite the smaller payoffs and the greater degree of work needed to obtain them[§§].

Another way that providers can protect themselves from litigation is by avoiding the higher risk situations

§§ Why is it that when an individual carries no medical insurance he is called "uninsured", but when a physician carries no malpractice insurance he is called "self-insured"?

inherent to their field. The classic example of this is the emergency room, the most litigious environment in which a physician can practice his trade. This factor, coupled with the often onerous lifestyle restrictions and poor payer mix, strongly motivates physicians to discontinue providing emergency room services thus compounding the manpower shortage.

Early retirement is an option that is becoming increasingly viable to the aging physician population. Many are considering this as the ultimate method of curtailing their practice risk. These generally are physicians who could easily practice five to ten more years and are seeking ways to restructure their debt and alter their lifestyles to accommodate the lower income levels that not practicing would afford them.

Other physicians, particularly younger ones, consider moving to lower-risk states rather than continuing to practice in higher-risk ones. The classic example of a state benefiting from alleviating its medical malpractice situation is Texas. Since 2004, when Texas imposed its constitutional amendment serving to cap medical malpractice awards, this state has witnessed an 18 percent increase in the number of medical licenses issued. The overall effect has been to elevate Texas from 48th in per capita physician concentration to 42nd with an associated 21.3 percent drop in medical malpractice insurance premiums.[36]

Texas's experience demonstrates another method that can be employed to lower the risk to the practicing provider-- tort reform. Approximately 35 states have implemented some form of cap on medical malpractice awards.[36] These measures have had varying effects on curbing malpractice premiums and promoting more favorable practice environments depending largely on the severity of their restrictions

CHAPTER 3:

THE BAUCUS PLAN

What is the Baucus Plan?

Senator Max Baucus (D-MT) is the chairman of Senate Finance Committee. His position affords him great influence in the shaping of any legislation relating to health care reform. On November 12, 2008, he released a white paper entitled "Call to Action-Health Reform 2009," in which he summarizes his vision for health care reform in this country. Available for review in PDF format at http://finance.senate.gov/healthreform2009/finalwhitepaper.pdf, the report presents a working framework for the creation of an American health care system that would provide affordable, high-quality health care to all Americans. "Call to Action", or The Baucus Plan as the Senator refers to it, is of particular significance not only because it is being forwarded by the chairman of the Senate Finance Committee, but because it complies with the ideals and philosophies of the ranking members of the Democrat Party and is designed to mesh with President Barack Obama's plans for the creation of a universal health care model for this country. It is also similar to the ideals upheld by the Secretary of Health and Human Services nominee, Mr. Thomas Daschle. The Baucus Plan therefore, represents the leading framework for any attempt at health care reform.

Julio Gonzalez, M.D.

Considering that health care reform is sure to be one of the pivotal legislative endeavors of the upcoming Congress, it is imperative that the Baucus Plan be scrupulously studied not only by health care providers and members of the health care industry, but also by all Americans, as any plan that is drawn up by the legislature will have a direct bearing on the way each of us receives our care and how it will be funded.

The Framework of the Baucus Plan

As mentioned previously, the goal of the Baucus Plan is to construct a national health care system that allows all inhabitants of the United States to receive high-quality, affordable health care independent of age, race, ethnicity, or income.[37] Stated differently, under the Baucus Plan, if you find yourself inside the United States, you should benefit from the national health care system regardless of who you are, how you got here, or your ability to pay. Additionally, the level and sophistication of care that you get, whether it be a life-saving measure or a purely elective intervention, should not vary regardless of who you are, how you got here, or your ability to pay.

Although there is little doubt over the appropriateness of equal access to health care regardless of one's ethnicity, age, or gender, the concept of one's income or ability to pay and the legitimacy of one's presence in this country not serving as factors in accessing care is far from being universally accepted. Despite this, the Baucus Plan supports the contention for universal health care by citing the United States as the only developed country "without health coverage to all of its citizens." [38]

Adhering to such a criterion in ensuring health care coverage for our population would mean that not only will those Americans who are poor and unable to pay for their own health care benefit from such a system, the 11.8 million people who find themselves in the United States illegally would also be eligible for participation. In either case, whether here illegally or unable to fund one's own health care through one's own means, the result of this philosophical outlook on health care availability is that those who are earning greater compensation and are able to fund their own care will be funding the care for those who can't as well as those who won't.

The logic behind this philosophical position is derived from the belief that universal involvement in the health care delivery system will result in more affordable health care to all individuals. According to this belief, the 46 million uninsured (15.3 percent of the population) and 25 million underinsured living in the United States have the net effect of driving up health care prices, as providers and organizations strive to make up for the costs of providing uncompensated care. It is felt that if the whole population were funded, there would be no financial strain from uncompensated or undercompensated care and the prices of providing care would fall. These lower prices would then be passed on to the insurance consumer by way of lower premiums. Additionally, since a larger segment of the population would be paying for their care while still healthy, their contributions to the health care insurance fund would serve to lower insurance premiums.

The Baucus Plan is based on three principles that serve as the foundation for the legislative effort: 1) every American should have health coverage, 2) the cost of health care delivery must be lowered, and 3) health care is a shared responsibility of every American*. In order to achieve these goals, the Baucus Plan relies on a three-pronged attack to the problem: 1) improving access to affordable health care coverage, 2) reforming the health care delivery system so as to improve value, and 3) promoting the development of a more efficient health care system. These will be discussed in detail.

---

* In his report Senator Baucus does not specify who shares this respon-sibility. I used Americans, because this is the segment of the population to which our legislative structure applies, but as will be explained later, there are inconsistencies throughout "Call to Action" over whether the Senator feels this responsibility is shared by all Americans or all inhabitants.

Improving Access

Under the Baucus Plan, it will be everyone's responsibility to obtain health care coverage. Health care coverage will be mandated.

The Baucus Plan will depend on a strong, employer-based insurance coverage system. Tasking the employer with providing insurance for his employees will be associated with lower administrative costs, as each plan would cover a group of individuals, not just one. All except the smallest businesses would offer a mandatory Section 125 plan* that would include health care insurance. The larger companies, especially those paying higher wages, will contribute at higher rates. Those companies that choose not to provide health care coverage for their employees but are capable of doing so will be required to make contributions to a fund designed to implement coverage for those who are unable to pay. The contribution would be based on the size and annual revenues of each firm. Small businesses would be provided with a tax credit to fund the purchase of health insurance for their employees and would be exempt from

---

*　　Section 125 plans, or cafeteria plans, are funds in which employers may participate that allow the employees to allocate pre-tax contributions to certain benefits such as health insurance.

the responsibility of covering their employees if they are unable to do so. Individuals and families at the lower income brackets would also receive subsidies that would allow them to afford health care coverage.

Additionally, public health care programs such as Medicare, Medicaid, Children's Health Insurance Program (CHIP), and the Indian Health Service (IHS) would be strengthened. While the Plan is being phased-in, individuals between the ages of 55 and 65 would be afforded the opportunity to buy into Medicare. This option would be eliminated over a few years as the provisions of universal health care are implemented. The Baucus Plan would also serve to strengthen the role of Medicaid by mandating that all states make everyone living at or below poverty level eligible for care. The federal government would help achieve this end by increasing its Federal Medical Assistance Package to the states with even further contributions being made during times of economic hardship.[†]

Access to affordable health care coverage will be guaranteed through a health insurance Exchange. The Exchange will "organize affordable health insurance options, create understandable, comparable information about those options, and develop a standard application for enrollment in a chosen plan."[39]

An Independent Health Coverage Council would then be established, which essentially would function as a

---

† The Federal Medical Assistance Package is a financial support provided to the states by the federal government to assist the states in the maintenance of their Medicaid programs. This program offers states between a 50 and 83 percent match by federal funds for state Medicaid expenses. The percentage match is dependent on state per-capita income data.

board of governors. The council would make "informed decisions" that would help guarantee affordable health care. The members of the Health Coverage Council would be appointed by the President and approved by the Senate and would be responsible for defining coverage and affordability. The Council would be tasked with managing such variables as expenses, establishing out-of-pocket costs, setting quality standards and cost effectiveness requirements, and mandating the type and quality of care delivered.

The Baucus Plan would prohibit insurance companies from denying coverage for individuals with preexisting conditions. Rules would be established determining how much insurance companies can manipulate their charges based on high-risk conditions or lifestyles, such as smoking, previous illness, or other factors.

In order to help facilitate the delivery of preventive medicine services, a "Right Choices" card would be created. This card would allow the uninsured access to preventive medicine services such as health risk assessment, physical exams, immunizations, and cancer screenings recommended by the U.S. Preventive Services Task Force. Each patient would be given a care plan designed to help maintain good health. The Right Choices card would also provide referrals to community resources such as smoking cessation and nutrition programs. If an individual with a Right Choices card is identified as having a medical condition that can be treated or prevented and is not otherwise insured, the patient would then be eligible for treatment of that condition. Of course, these interventions would only be needed until the Health Insurance Exchange becomes operational at which time a more permanent form of coverage would become available. Communities would be "empowered and encouraged to identify and overcome barriers to healthy choices for all residents, regardless of health status, race or socioeconomic status."[40]

Improving Value

More funding would be provided for the primary physician and emphasis would be placed on a medical home model. The viability of community care centers and rural health clinics would also be assured. The medical infrastructure would be modernized through the improvement of health information technology (IT) so that health care providers would have better access to unbiased information and clinical support tools.

A pay-for-performance program, such as the one instituted by Medicare, would be emphasized. Such models can be expanded to include nursing homes and health care facilities. Similarly, pay-for-reporting programs such as those instituted in hospitals by Medicare would also be studied for expansion. These basic programs of reporting and accountability would then be elevated to quality-based reimbursement programs that would essentially link the care delivered to the achievement of quality goals, a concept named value-based purchasing.

Physician performance would also be more meticulously reviewed. The Physicians Quality Reporting Initiative (PQRI) is a Medicare program that tasks physicians with reporting information relating to certain care measures. The system allows Congress to receive information about the quality of care provided. It also allows for the documentation of information that can be shared between physicians. Medical registries are banks of information documenting patient treatment and their outcomes.

The Baucus Plan aims to foster these programs and then link PQRI with the medical boards' maintenance-of-certifications process. Consequently, physicians would no longer be required only to take conventional tests once every ten years in order to maintain their certification, but to incorporate quality and outcomes reporting as an integral part of the test-taking process. More frequent recertification requirements would also be required. These would include patient testimonials and patients reporting data about physicians.

Another method for improving quality that could be instituted is the per-capita resource use. Here, physicians are evaluated based on the amount of resources they are using on the treatment of patients with particular conditions. Third-party payers would then be able to identify physicians whose practice habits fall outside of the average by way of the amount of resources they employ on a particular condition. In so doing, the third-party payer may then work to incentivize, or pressure, the targeted physician with the aim of streamlining, or diminishing the amount of resources employed on a particular condition. Data on the use of resources expended per episode would be collected and made available to third-party payers.

Private plans that participate in Medicare would also be asked to participate in quality review. The

Medicare Advantage plans would therefore be included in this effort of reporting quality.

The Baucus Plan also calls for the repair of the Sustainable Growth Rate formula for physician reimbursement. As previously illustrated, the formula is fundamentally flawed and has consistently called for cuts in physician reimbursement rates since 2002. These cuts have been unrealistic and have consistently been reversed by congressional action. The payment scheme would be abandoned or extensively modified while concentrating on formulas that remove expenditure target goals but promote quality-based reimbursement schemes and/or geographical or types-of-service-measures as drivers of the targets for reimbursement. The modified SGR would then be employed to emphasize certain treatment methods and approaches while de-emphasizing others.

As costs are lowered, health care provider groups would reap the rewards from any expense reductions through gain sharing, a process by which physicians are reimbursed for any cost savings they may have realized.

Financing a More Efficient Health Care System

It is estimated that funding for a universal health care system would result in anywhere from $100 billion to $150 billion in new federal spending.[41] In order to keep the program budget neutral, this extra financing burden would be offset by savings obtained from streamlining the health care system and improving its efficiency. Although the previously named interventions are predicted to help reduce the costs of administering health care, further steps will be needed to curb excess spending. Initiatives would be implemented to curtail fraud, waste, and abuse. Competitive bidding programs would be instituted as would vigilant government oversight. Strong punishments for those who try to defraud the system would also be implemented. Increased reporting of the costs and quality of health care delivered will be required as well as details regarding the nature of relationships between industry and health care providers. Physician self-referral would be strongly resisted and prosecuted. Hospital ownership would be prohibited. Medical malpractice laws would be revised. Overpayment to private Medicare insurance providers would be eliminated. New models would be developed in order to help diminish the costs of long-term health services. Tax reforms would be explored with the aim of reducing health care spending.

In conclusion, the Baucus Plan as summarized in "Call to Action" would aim to pervade every element of the health care system, from coverage specifications, to the micromanagement of practice standards, to the rationing of care and manipulation of the models through which health care is delivered. The central driving force would be seeking methods and structures that benefit the government and society, and not necessarily the individual patient.

CHAPTER 4:

MISCONCEPTIONS

Universal Access Versus
Universal Coverage

Many promoters of health care reform cite the need for "universal health care". They say it is "inexcusable" for people living in the United States not to have access to health care. This derogatory depiction of our willingness to care for the poor and destitute is inherently false. As already noted, *everyone* in this country, whether here legally or not, has access to health care. What we are really debating is the degree of mandated health care *coverage* that we want and the extent to which taxpayers should be held accountable for that coverage. We have already decided that people with life or limb threatening conditions should have access to care. The true question then is to what extent should society support health care for other than urgent or emergent conditions and should the afflicted individual be held financially accountable for the cost of his care regardless of his socioeconomic status.

Julio Gonzalez, M.D.

The True Scope of Uninsurance

Proponents of health care reform claim there are 46 million uninsured individuals living in the United States, or 13.5 percent of the population. However, as previously noted this 46 million includes the 11.8 million individuals estimated to be living in this country illegally. Most Americans oppose the public financing of health care services for unauthorized inhabitants.[19,42] The 46 million figure also includes 17.6 million people who can afford health care insurance, but opt not to purchase it, representing another segment of the population for whom most feel unmotivated to publicly fund care. Consequently, a more honest assessment of the number of people on whom we should be focusing our efforts at providing assistance with their health care coverage is that segment of the population that is living legitimately in the United States and is either unable to get appropriate health insurance coverage or is having great difficulty in obtaining it. At the very most, this number comprises the 16.3 million legitimate inhabitants of the United States who are either poor or members of the lower middle class, plus the segment of the approximately 1.3 million people who are "uninsurable" and also members of these two lower socioeconomic strata. These two groups account for a maximum total of about 17.6 million people.

The United States Is the Only Developed Country That Does Not Provide Health Coverage for All Its Citizens

Absolutely not true. The Central Intelligence Agency in its *The World Factbook* categorizes countries according to their economic development.[43] Developed countries generally have a per-capita gross domestic product of greater than $10,000. These countries are considered to be the most advanced in the world and are also known as "the first world." They are listed in Table 4.1. Within this group South Africa and Bermuda do not provide universal health care, thus nullifying the validity of the claim. Additionally, a number of other countries that are claimed to provide universal health care require individuals to register with the government in order to be eligible for health care services. If one is a citizen of a European country, then proof of citizenship is required prior to receiving care. Individuals who are not citizens of participating European countries are required to obtain a European Health Insurance Card in order to gain access to non-emergent services. Regardless of the degree of universality being ascribed to these countries, they generally do not provide elective health care services for individuals residing illegally in that country.

Additionally, it may not even be appropriate to place the United States in the same demographic and historical category as other members of the developed world. Except for Israel, Canada, and South Africa, all 35 developed countries arose from monarchies or serfdoms. This is of great significance in terms of the design of their respective health care systems. These countries arose from a national model where the government (the king or monarch) was responsible for taking care of its subjects. As time went on, these countries generally gravitated away from totalitarianism and toward a more democratic system of government. It would therefore be historically logical for these nations to design health care systems under the umbrella of their new governments, as the concept of significant government involvement in the day-to-day dealings of the citizenry is ingrained into their cultures.

The United States arrived at its present position through a radically different approach. America developed out of a need to flee the effects of totalitarianism and religious oppression. From the moment its people first set foot on this continent their every fiber was bent on resisting oppression and governmental authority. What's more, no single nationalistic group was able to establish itself as the overwhelming majority. The different groups coalesced, seeking ways of working together toward a common goal, initially of survival, later of subsistence, and finally of excelling. The American people did not break from a single government or monarchy, but rather it tamed a continent while fighting lawlessness and ethnic friction throughout its plight. As such, it would be naïve to imply, as seems to be the case by the proponents of universal health care reform, that all the developed countries are right in providing universal health care and the United States is somehow the final holdout. Rather, the different system designs are lasting footprints of each country's national development and historical experience. If anything, the trend is for those countries still upholding single-payer, universal health care schemes to move increasingly away from a centralized system and toward one that allows for greater independence.

Julio Gonzalez, M.D.

The United States Health Care System Is Not the Best in the World

This point is *highly* disputable. In 2000, the United Nations' World Health Organization delivered its final list of rankings of national health care systems. First among these was France. The United States was ranked 37th, just two places above Cuba.[44] This paltry showing, with a price tag numbering in the trillions, is noted as evidence for the inefficiency of the American health care system. However, even a cursory analysis of this claim calls its validity into serious contention.

In a virtual acknowledgement of the inconsistencies of their rankings, the WHO discontinued ranking health care systems in 2000 because of the complexity of the task and inaccuracy of their data collection process, thus acknowledging the shortcomings of its methodologies. One of these flaws is assigning the United States a lower ranking simply because it does not possess a funded universal health care system. Consequently, irrespective of the sophistication or complexity of the American health care system, the mere fact that universal health care coverage is not an integral part of its design will cause it to appear lower in the rankings than it deserves. On the other hand, countries with deplorable health care systems such as Communist Cuba where there is widespread shortage of supplies and a lack of cleanliness of its facilities will score higher. Other factors that are multi-factorial in influence such as longevity, infant mortality and obesity rates are also considered in determining the final rankings. These factors may serve more as testaments to a population's lifestyle and dietary conditions than reflections of the efficacy of its health care system, but is nevertheless given a significant amount of weight.

Table 4.1 lists the countries that rank above the United States according to the WHO.[44] One immediately realizes that comparisons to the majority of these countries are at best invalid. For starters, the average population of the countries ranking above the United States is 20,287,309, approximately 7 percent of the United States population[43]. The closest population to that of the United States is Japan, with a population of 127,288,416, or 42 percent that of the United States. It is a lot easier to provide care for a smaller group of people than it is to provide it to upwards of 300 million. A look at the rankings of countries that are similar or larger in population to the United States exemplifies the point. Brazil, with a population of 196,342, 592, ranks 125th. Russia with a population of 140,702,096, ranks 130th. China, with a population of 1,330,044,544, ranks 144th. Pakistan, India, and Indonesia, with populations of 172,800,048, 1,147,995,904 and 237,512,352 respectively, rank 122nd, 112th and 92nd. The conclusion is that whether it is due to the economic strain placed on a country by its sheer size or the logistical considerations associated with delivering care to such a large group of people, countries with a higher number of inhabitants have a much more difficult time establishing a health care system that would rank well in the WHO ranking scale. Interestingly, of the large countries considered, only the United States and Japan are afforded reasonable rankings.

Country	WHO Ranking	Population
France	1	64,057,792
Italy	2	58,145,320
San Marino	3	29,973
Andorra	4	86,627
Malta	5	403,532
Singapore	6	4,608,167
Spain	7	40,491,052
Oman	8	3,311,640
Austria	9	8,205,533
Japan	10	127,288,416
Norway	11	4,644,457
Portugal	12	10,676,910
Monaco	13	32,796
Greece	14	10,722,816
Iceland	15	304,367
Luxembourg	16	486,006
Netherlands	17	16,645,313
United Kingdom	18	60,943,912
Ireland	19	4,156,119
Switzerland	20	7,581,520
Belgium	21	10,403,951
Colombia	22	45,013,672
Sweden	23	9,045,389
Cyprus	24	792,604
Germany	25	82,369,552
Saudi Arabia	26	28,146,656
United Arab Emirates	27	4,621,399
Israel	28	7,112,359
Morocco	29	34,343,220
Canada	30	33,212,696
Finland	31	5,244,749
Australia	32	21,007,310
Chile	33	16,454,143
Denmark	34	5,484,723
Dominica	35	72,514
Costa Rica	36	4,195,914
United States of America	37	303,824,640
Mean Population Excluding U.S.		20,287,308.86

Table 4.1 World Health Organization Rankings for Health Care per Capita Spending

73

The High Infant Mortality Rate

As noted in Table 4.2, the United States' infant mortality rate is higher than any of its western European counterparts of the developed world. At 6.3 deaths per thousand live infants, however, it is not the highest in the developed world, as the Faroe Islands (6.46), Bermuda (7.87), Russia (10.81), Turkey (36.98), and South Africa (45.11) carry higher rates. According to "Call to Action", the infant mortality rate in the United States is almost double that of France and Germany.[2] The same source observes that the infant mortality rate of African Americans is higher than that of Slovenia, Poland, Kuwait, and Russia.[45] However, as we will see, the use of this statistic in an effort to discredit the American health care system is arguably *the* most intellectually dishonest use of a statistic in the health care reform debate.

The infant mortality rate (IMR) is the number of babies per 1,000 live babies born each year that die during the first year of life. The statistic is used as a guide in obtaining a gross idea of the state of a region's health care. As one might guess, a myriad of prenatal and postnatal factors influence the rate at which babies die during the first year of life. These include factors that are directly related to health care delivery efficiency such as access to and quality of a mother's prenatal care, as well as access to and the quality of the baby's care during its first year of life. Other factors influenced by quality of health care include prematurity rates and average birth weights. However, a number of other factors not related to health care quality influence the IMR. These include maternal behaviors, lifestyle decisions, substance abuse problems, nutritional problems, prenatal smoking habits, the presence of chronic illnesses, the position in which the baby is placed to sleep, the firmness of the mattress, whether the child sleeps by himself or with others, how much the child is fed, the baby's body fat percentage, and even the number of toys with which a child sleeps. Consequently, although the IMR can serve as a gross estimate of a region's health care system, with so many cultural and non health care related influences, it cannot be used to compare health care system qualities among countries with similar infant mortality rates.

However, this uncertainty by itself is insufficient at reflecting the degree of deceit with which the IMR is being employed in public policy debates. The significance of a region's infant mortality rates cannot be fully understood without accounting for fetal mortality rates. The fetal mortality rate is the number of babies that die in utero before being born. Inclusive of this number is the subgroup of babies who may have been born with some signs of life and not resuscitated per protocol or policy. Obviously, regional variations on what constitutes a live birth have a tremendous impact on the reported infant mortality rate for each respective region. Stated another way, if a baby is born "practically" dead but meets criteria for an attempt at resuscitation, and the resuscitation effort is initially successful but the baby goes on to die, that death is listed as an infant death, thus boding poorly for that country's infant mortality rate. However, if that same baby were to be born in a country of less sophistication and the delivery team does not attempt a resuscitation, then that baby would be listed as a "stillborn" and registered as a fetal death. It would therefore not count as an infant death and consequently not impact the infant mortality rate at all. It is this discrepancy in reporting that gives the United States, with its incredibly advanced, incredibly expensive, and incredibly aggressive neonatal units a falsely elevated infant mortality rate. The question is…where would you rather deliver your baby?

The United States uses the WHO definition of live birth when reporting its infant mortality rate:

> *"Live birth refers to the complete expulsion or extraction from its mother of a product of conception, irrespective of the duration of the pregnancy, which, after such separation, breathes or shows any other evidence of life - e.g. beating of the heart, pulsation of the umbilical cord or definite movement of voluntary muscles - whether or not the umbilical cord has been cut or the placenta is attached. Each product of such a birth is considered live born."*[46]

Although this is the criterion recommended by the WHO, it is not universally employed, even in developed countries. In the United Kingdom, live birth registration of babies that did not show any signs of life are limited to those that are born after 24 weeks of gestational age. Their criteria do not address babies born prior to 24 weeks of age. France's guidance on this issue is even less descriptive, relying on a certificate that attests that the child was born "alive and viable". The Netherlands do not resuscitate children below 25 weeks of gestational age, and Switzerland uses only respirations and heart beat as their criteria for live birth.[47]

In the United States, babies born at less than 24 weeks of gestational age (six months of pregnancy) are routinely resuscitated and attempted to be kept alive provided they have any signs of life at the time of birth. Some of these babies weigh less than 500 grams (1.10 pounds). As could be imagined, these "extremely low birth weight babies" have a much higher complication rate following birth, and predictably, a much higher death rate during the first year of life. Yet, each of these babies is cared for in the United States, one of a very elite number of countries that can even make the attempt. Each of these baby's deaths count against the United States' infant mortality rate, only to be used against it by individuals, many of them politicians, who are out to discredit the sophistication of our health care system.

What kind of an impact do these differences in resuscitation philosophy have on infant mortality rates? In 2005, 12.7 percent of births in the United States were preterm (less than 37 weeks gestational age) and 2.03 percent were very preterm (less than 32 weeks gestational age).[48,49] Approximately 68.6 percent of infant deaths in the United States occurred in preterm children while very preterm infants accounted for 2 percent of infant deaths.[48] These numbers have increased since 2000.

Ironically, another factor that seems to be playing a negative role in increasing the very low weight birth rate, and in turn the infant mortality rate, is the higher incidence of pregnancies achieved through assisted reproductive technologies. Women who undergo these infertility treatments tend to be older and have a higher incidence of multiple gestations. The United States has been a leader in the development and delivery of infertility technology, another example of an area where the advances of the American health care system are working against its infant mortality figures.

Although no epidemiologist can deny the discrepancies in infant survival data between different racial and ethnic groups within the United States, only comparisons of relative mortality data measured within the United States have any chance of carrying any validity. Any comparison of our statistical experience in neonatal health care with that of any other country is scientifically invalid and has no role in the health care policy debate except to discredit its proponent.

COUNTRY	FOUNDED	GOVERNMENT TYPE	POPULATION	MEAN AGE (YRS)	OLDER THAN 64 (%)	POPULATION GROWTH RATE (%)	NET MIGRATION RATE (MIGRANTS PER 1000)	LIFE EXPECTANCY AT BIRTH (YRS)	INFANT MORTALITY RATE (PER THOUSAND)	GDP (BILLION DOLLARS)	GDP PER CAPITA	POVERTY RATE (%)	UNEMPLOYMENT RATE (%)	HEALTH CARE SYSTEM	HEALTH CARE % GDP	WHO RANKING*
Andorra	1278	I	82,627	38.9	12	0.019	13.99	82.67	NA	2.77	38,800	Na^a	0	1,2,6,10	7.1	4
Australia	1901	II	21,007,310	37.1	13.3	0.012	6.34	81.53	4.82	773	37,300	9.9^a,b	4.4	2,3,4,6,10	8.7	32
Austria	1955	III	8,205,533	41.7	17.5	0.064	1.88	79.36	4.48	322	39,300	5.9	4.4	3,7	10.3	9
Belgium	1830	II	10,403,951	41.4	17.5	0.106	1.22	79.02	4.5	376	36,200	15.2	7.5	2,3,10	10.3	21
Bermuda	NA	IV	66,536	41	12.8	0.546	2.28	78.3	7.87	4.5	69,900	19	2.1	3,8	3.3^j	Not Ranked
Canada	1867	VI	33,212,696	40.1	14.9	0.83	5.62	81.18	5.08	1,270,000	38,600	10.8	6	2,9,10	10	30
Denmark	965	VI	5,484,723	40.3	15.7	0.295	2.94	78.13	4.4	203.3	37,200		2.8	2,9,10	8.8^g	34
Faroe Islands	1948k	VII	46,668	36.7	14.1	0.376	-0.82	79.26	6.46		31,000		2.1	2,9,10	NA	Not Ranked
Finland	1917	VIII	5244749	41.8	16.6	0.112	0.73	78.82	3.5	188.4	36,000		6.9	2,9,10	8.2	31
France	486	VIII	57,792	39.2	16.3	0.574	1.48	80.87	3.36	2,0750,00	32,600	6.2	7.9	2,9,10	11	1
Germany	1990	III	82,369,552	43.4	20	-0.044	2.19	79.1	4.03	2,807,000	34,100		9	3,10	10.6	25
Greece	1974	IX	10,722,816	41.5	19.1	0.146	2.33	79.52	5.25	327.6	30,600	11	8.3	2,3,9,11	9.1	14
Holy See	1929	X	824	NA	NA	NA	NA	NA	NA	NA	NA	Na^a	NA	NA	NA	Not Ranked
Iceland	1944	XI	304,367	34.8	12	0.763	1.13	80.5	3.25	12.19	40,400		1	7-10p	9.1	15
Ireland	1921	I, VIII	4,156,159	34.6	11.8	1.133	4.76	78.07	5.14	191.6	46,600	7	4.6	2,3,9,10	7.5	19
Israel	1948	I	7,112,359	28.9	9.8	1.713	2.52	80.61	4.28	185.8	26,600	21.6	7.3	2,9,10	9	28
Italy	1861	VIII	58,145,320	42.9	20	-0.019	2.06	80.07	5.61	1,800,000	30,900		6.2	2,9,10	9	2

Table 4.2 Global Health Care Systems

COUNTRY	FOUNDED	GOVERNMENT TYPE	POPULATION	MEAN AGE (YRS)	OLDER THAN 64 (%)	POPULATION GROWTH RATE (%)	NET MIGRATION RATE (MIGRANTS PER 1000)	LIFE EXPECTANCY AT BIRTH (YRS)	INFANT MORTALITY RATE (PER THOUSAND)	GDP (BILLION DOLLARS)	GDP PER CAPITA	POVERTY RATE (%)	UNEMPLOYMENT RATE (%)	HEALTH CARE SYSTEM	HEALTH CARE % GDP	WHO RANKING*
Japan	660 BC	V,VI	127,288,416	43.8	21.6	-0.139	NA	82.07	2.8	4,272,000	33,500	15.3[a]	3.8	2,9,10	8.1	10
Liechtenstein	1866	VI	34,498	40.5	13.3	0.713	4.7	79.95	4.52	1.786	25,000	NA[a]	1.3	2,9,10	NA	Not Ranked
Luxembourg	1839	VI	486,606	39	14.7	1.188	8.54	79.18	4.62	38.14	79,400	4.4	4.4	2,9,10	7.3	16
Malta	1964	VIII	403,352	39.2	13.9	0.407	2.03	79.3	3.79	9.4	23,400	NA[a]	6.4	2,3	6.4[r]	5
Monaco	1338	VI	32,796	45.5	22.8	0.375	7.62	79.96	5.18	0.976	30,000	NA[a]	0	2,3	9.2[s]	13
Netherlands	1579	VI	16,645,313	40	14.6	0.436	2.55	79.25	4.81	645.5	39,000	NA[a]	4.6	2,3,	9.51	17
N Zealand	1907	I	4,173,460	36.3	12.6	0.971	2.62	80.24	4.99	112.4	27,200	10.4[a]	3.6	2.3,12	8.0[r]	41
Norway	1905	VI	4,644,457	39	15	0.35	1.71	79.81	3.61	346.6	53,300	6.3[a]	2.5	2,3,9,10	8.7	11
Portugal	1910	I, VIII	10,676,910	39.1	17.4	0.305	3.23	78.04	4.85	232.2	21,800	18	8	2,3,9	10.2	12
Russia	1991	XII	140,702,096	38.3	14.1	-0.474	0.28	65.94	10.81	2,097,000	14,800	15.8	6.2	2,9,11	2.6	130
San Marino	301	VIII	29,973	41.2	17.2	1.181	10.44	81.88	5.44	0.85	34,100	NA[a]	3.8	2,9	7.3[t]	3
S. Africa	1961	VIII	48,782,756	24.2	5.3	0.828	4.98	48.89	45.11	467.8	9,700	50	24.3	3,5,8	8.7	175
Spain	1492	V	40,491,052	40.7	17.9	0.096	0.99	79.92	4.26	1,361,000	33,600	19.8	8.3	2,3,9	8.4	7
Sweden	1523	VI	9,045,389	41.3	18.3	0.157	1.66	80.74	2.75	455.3	37,500	5.3[a]	6.1	2,3,9,10	9.2	23
Switzerland	1291	XIII	7,581,520	40.7	16	0.329	2.21	80.74	4.23	303.2	40,100	6.7	2.8	2,3,10	11.3	20
Turkey	1923	XIV	71,898,808	29	7	1.013	0	73.14	36.98	853.9	12,000	20	9.9	3	5.7[m]	70
UK	10th Century	XVI	60,943,912	39.9	16	0.276	2.17	78.85	4.93	2,130,000	35,000	14	5.3	2,3	8.4	18
US	1776	XV	303,824,640	36.7	12.7	0.883	2.92	78.14	6.3	13,780	45,800	12.5[c]	4.6	3,4,5,6	16.3	37

Table 4.2 Global Health Care Systems, cont.

a: CIA Factbook data not available
b: Source: theage.com
c: 4. U.S. Census Bureau, "Income, Poverty, and Health Insurance Coverage in the United States: 2007," U.S. Census Bureau,
d: Purchasing Power Parity
e: Source: Exxu.com
f: From CIA factbook unless otherwise stated.
g: OECD Database 2006
h: Source: Worldpress.org
i: Source: Indexmundi.com
j Source: paho.org (World Health Organization)
k: High degree of association with Denmark
l: OECD Database 2004
m: OECD Database 2005
n: OECD Database 2005
o: OECD Database 2005
p: No official estimates
q: Source: OECD(2004), Income Distribution and Poverty in OECD Countries in the Second Half of the 1990s.
r: Source: Central Office of Statistics Malta & Budgetary Estimates. 1996
s: Source: National Institute for Intelligence Studies. Mercyhurst College
t: Source: photius.com

* WHO discontinued ranking health care systems in 2000 because of inaccuracies in their methodologies.
1: Constitution guarantees health care rights.
2. Social health care system.
3. Public and private funding.
4. Public funding is split between federal and state sources
5. Routine health care coverage not guaranteed.
6. Although care not universal, emergent and urgent care guaranteed.
7. Social health care begins when an individual enters the workforce
8. Coverage not universal
9. Government funded, national health care system
10. Mandatory health insurance
11. Significant out of pocket expense from underground private activity due to dissatisfaction with public system
12. Primary health care partially funded. Specialty care and hospital stays publically funded

Government Types
I: Parliamentary democracy
II: Federal parliamentary democracy
III: Federal republic
IV: United Kingdom Territory
V Parliamentary monarchy
VI: Constitutional monarchy
VII: Self-Governing overseas division of Denmark
VIII: Republic
IX: Parliamentary republic
X: Ecclesiastical
XI: Constitutional republic
XII: Federation
XIII: Confederation
XIV: Republican parliamentary democracy
XV: Constitution based federal republic

Table 4.2 Global Health Care Systems, cont.

Is It the Uninsured Or Is It the Poor?

"…the plight of the uninsured is unconscionable."— Secretary Designee of the Department of Health and Human Services Designee, Thomas Daschle, December 11, 2008.

It is interesting that Secretary Designee Mr. Thomas Daschle should use the term "plight" to describe the difficulties of being uninsured in America since the term is usually used to discuss the reality of life in poverty ("the plight of the poor"). The obvious intent of using this term in reference to the uninsured is to somehow equate the challenges of being uninsured with the hardships of poverty. This, of course, is disingenuous considering that many of the uninsured in this country are facing no rigors at all. There is no plight if you are healthy, do not get hurt, and have no medical insurance. There is similarly no plight if you are rich and choose not to purchase medical insurance. However, people who are poor almost universally have a "plight". Where will they get their food? How will they keep the roof over their heads? How will they afford their medicines? Those are the hardships with which those living in poverty struggle regardless of whether they have health insurance or not. On the other hand, the only people without health insurance who are confronted with a plight are those who have little or no money and develop a pressing health care problem.

It's a matter of identifying the real malady behind the problem. Suppose that the primary cause of a population's health disparity is their economic status and not their insurance status. If this is the case, then improving the population's health care coverage rate will accomplish very little towards the goal of affording it better health. Improving its economic condition, on the other hand, might.

A significant amount of evidence exists suggesting that poverty is the major contributor to a country's health disparity, not a lack of health insurance coverage.[50] The Joint Canada/United States Survey of Health provides insight into the relative contributions of uninsurance and poverty to the health of a population.[51] This report demonstrated mirrored variations among the economic strata in both Canada and the United States with the United States scoring somewhat worse in most indices. Although the authors felt that universal health care afforded better health indices, cultural differences between the two populations can also explain the noted variations. More important was the finding that in Canada, where funded health care is afforded to all, the same association between poverty and poor health was preserved, suggesting that the underlying malady leading to the symptom of poor health in a population is poverty, not necessarily uninsurance.

The Government Can Deliver Health Care At a Significantly Lower Cost Than the Private Sector

With the countless examples of governmental inefficiency and waste, it is perplexing that the claim of the relative efficiency of government health care delivery would be promoted as accurate. Nevertheless, it is one of the most frequently touted reasons for promoting a single-payer, government-run, health care system. It is difficult to pinpoint the origin of this misconception, but it seems to be at least partly based on data produced by the National Health Expenditures (NHE) account report.[52,53] According to the 2005 data released in this report, Medicare's administrative costs run about 3.1 percent of total health care spending (7.0 percent for Medicaid). This compares to the 14.1 percent in the case of private insurance companies touted in this report, or the 25 percent that is commonly espoused.

However, the NHE figures are deficient. A review of the NHE data reveals a number of cost categories included in the private sector date, but not considered for Medicare. These include tax collection costs to fund Medicare (analogous to premium collection costs by private insurers), marketing, outreach and education costs, customer service costs, program auditing costs for work done by the Office of the Inspector General, contract negotiation costs, building costs, staff salaries for CMS personnel with Medicare program responsibilities, and Congressional resources exhausted on setting Medicare payment rates for services.[54] Costs included in the private sector analysis that do not apply to government funded programs include taxes paid.

Once these true but hidden expenses are noted, the administrative costs of Medicare funded health care approaches those encountered in the private sector. In an analysis performed by Mark Litow and the Council for Affordable Health Insurance, the government was found to spend 66 percent more to provide health care coverage than private insurance.[55] In a more recent follow-up paper, estimates for the true administrative costs of health care delivery by Medicare amount to about 6 to 8 percent.[56] Adjusting for the private sector's costs for taxes and commissions brings the administrative costs of private insurance plans to about 8.9 percent, thus nullifying the argument of government-run health care posing a distinct cost advantage over its private sector competitors.

There are two other factors that although difficult to quantify tip the scales in favor of private insurance. The first is that some of the administrative costs incurred by private insurers are not wasteful because they are designed to help minimize costs in some other segment of their product. As an example, an administrative cost investment of one percent to help curtail a 10 percent strain from fraud and abuse would not be considered wasteful and would result in an overall expenditure savings of nine percent.

The second is mathematically more concrete and arises from the higher expense per claim associated with Medicare funded health care. Since Medicare pays much higher costs per claim because of the sicker state of the elderly population to which it is responsible, these higher total costs would make the administrative costs seem less as a percentage of the total costs of health care delivery. This influence is not a testament of Medicare's efficiency, but rather the effect of the higher amounts it has to spend in paying for the health care services it delivers.[57]

CHAPTER 5:

WHERE ARE THE STAKEHOLDERS (PROVIDERS AND PATIENTS)?

The Baucus Plan may have been doomed even before the first letter of the document was etched onto the senator's hard drive due to the notable absence of active health care provider participation.

The membership of the Senate Finance Committee, the team charged with playing the lead role in the development of any health care legislation, includes no physicians, chiropractors, nurses, nurse's aides, physical therapists, podiatrists, or dietitians. With the exception of Doctor and Senator John Ensign (R NV), who is a veterinarian, there is no member who has any direct experience in providing health care...to *any* species.[58] As a result, the major players in the development of any health care reform have little insight into the day-to-day dealings of a medical office, hospital, or clinic. Indeed, of the 21 members of the Senate Finance Committee, 10 (47 percent) are attorneys, four (19 percent) have degrees in political science or social-related studies, one (5 percent) is a retired baseball player, one (5 percent) is a farmer, one (5 percent) is a journalist, one (5 percent) is an engineer, one (5 percent) is a veterinarian, one (5 percent) is a social worker, and one (5 percent) is a computer software executive.

What's worse, the people from whom their ideas are sought are also lacking in direct patient-interaction experience. In his introductory letter to "Call to Action Health Care Reform 2009," Senator Baucus notes that much of his insight and work into the design of the Baucus Plan emanates from the nine hearings on health care held by the Senate Finance Committee during 2008.[59] A review of the public testimonies taken during the nine hearings before this committee demonstrate a general paucity of practicing health care providers. Of the 43 witnesses called before the committee, only eight were physicians, and of these, two were chief medical officers for insurance companies, one was the chief executive officer of the American Board of Medical Specialties, one was the dean of a medical school, one was the chief executive officer of a major health care system, and one was a member of the Urban Institute.[60,61,62,63,64,65,66,67,68,69,70,71,72]   Indeed there was a concerted effort by the senator to avoid the participation of the American Medical Association, the country's leading physician advocacy group.[73] The National Medical Association, representatives of the different medical specialty societies, representatives of the state medical societies, the American Hospital Association, the American Nursing Association, the American Chiropractic Association, the American Podiatric Association, the American Physical Therapy Association also lacked any representation in these testimonies. There was therefore no insight obtained about the challenges faced by rank-and-file health care providers in delivering care, nor was there any input from these direct stakeholders on improving the health care system and the process of providing care to patients.

The same personnel allocation error is encountered in the Senate Health, Education, Labor and Pensions Committee where of the 20 members, 10 are attorneys, one is a veterinarian, and only one is a physician. The only other physician serving in the Senate is not a member of any of the jurisdictional committees on health care.[74]

This crucial error is not unique to the Senate. The Medicare Payment Advisory Commission, the primary body responsible for advising Congress about legislative and policy issues related to health care is chaired by…you guessed it…a lawyer[75]. The vice chair holds a masters degree in public administration. Of the 16 members in MedPAC, only four carry degrees in medicine.[76] And let's not forget President Clinton's Task Force on National Health Care Reform, headed by Mrs. Clinton (also a lawyer). This secretive clan of policy-making consultants to the First Lady, and ultimately the President, consisted of 511 members; not a single one was a physician.[77]

This elemental flaw to the Baucus Plan is one that will not be encountered within its pages, but *is* one that is clearly felt. Dispersed throughout the Plan are assumptions regarding the flaws of health care delivery and its shortcomings that are based on academic studies and think-tank philosophies that do not necessarily reflect the experiences of those engaged in the field. If anything, it is the health care provider who should be charting up the plans for the health care delivery system and the health policy expert, economist and lawyer serving as his consultants and advisers.

CHAPTER 6:

MANIPULATION OF THE MARKET

The Baucus Plan and the modern health care reform movement are predicated on the notion that the market is inept at ensuring the adequacy of health care delivery. The free market, with its propensity for abuse, cannot control the opportunistic forces that drive its players. Only the government, with its sage and learned members, is able to place a calming effect on the market allowing everyone to benefit from its presence. The health care industry is therefore one to be thoroughly regulated ensuring that health care is delivered appropriately to all corners of our society.

These principles inherent to the modern health care reform movement run counter to the mercantilistic forces that helped build this country, but they pervade every aspect of the health care reform plans.

Julio Gonzalez, M.D.

The Health Insurance Exchange

In "Call to Action," as well as in the vision for
health care reform promoted by President Barack Obama,
a concerted effort is made to strengthen the employer's
role in the funding and administration of the health care
system. This type of willful shift of the health care market
structure represents the first and most elemental of a series
of measures designed to impose the government's will
on the free market and the Health Insurance Exchange
is the medium through which the manipulation will be
effected.

The Insurance Exchange, as described in "Call to
Action" is a network of insurance plans and companies
administered and mandated by the government designed
to task the employer with the responsibility of funding
and maintaining the health care system for all non-elderly
individuals living in the United States.[78] This flies in the
face of the stated foundation of "individual responsibility"
on which the Baucus Plan claims to be based, as it
diverges the burden for funding and administering
health care coverage away from the individual and to the
employer and government. Under this mandated strategy,
there is no room for individual responsibility because
health care coverage is legally required and provided

to everyone whether they choose to contribute to it or not. Since the burden of owning insurance coverage is government mandated and employer or publicly funded, the only responsibility for health care coverage left to the individual is a legal one. The "responsibility" referred to under the Baucus Plan, therefore, applies only to a legal one-meaning that under the Baucus Plan, the individual will be prosecuted and punished for not having procured some form of health care coverage.

Placing more weight on an employer may not be a truly sage plan. Let us start by acknowledging that the employer-based health care stake in this country arose not through social design, but as the result of a historical accident. In World War II, the government imposed wage freezes on American workers. In response, employers began offering health care coverage and other benefits as a way to attract better employees. Even though the concept of employer-based health care coverage eventually took root and formed the basis of an employee benefits network that supplies 59 percent of the coverage for non-elderly individuals living in the United States, it was never intended to fulfill some need of delivering health care coverage to the masses.

The most obvious disadvantage associated with employer-based health care insurance is that of restricting the individual's choice of insurance coverage as it is the employer and not the individual who gets to select the plan.[79] Additionally, because of the lack of portability, the employee is often forced to pick between his job and his preferred health insurance coverage. Because most plans carry a preexisting conditions clause restricting payment for health conditions that were present prior to enrolling

99

in the plan, making a change in employment can often result in a 6- to 12-months interruption in the care of a chronic health condition. Additionally, since the patient's physician may not participate in the new insurance plan, changes in employment can also result in the severing of perfectly favorable patient-doctor relationships.

Tasking the employer with providing a greater share of the insurance burden will have significant implications on the nation's economic health as well. As larger companies strive to meet the demands of contributing to the Exchange, cost-containment strategies will be instituted, including wage reductions and layoffs. The predictable effect will be to slow the economy, increase unemployment and diminish mean wage earnings, all of which serve to increase the national poverty rate resulting in a direct detrimental effect on health care.

In addition, there is reason to believe that employer-based plans may no longer serve as an effective way of addressing our country's health care delivery challenges.[80] Employees are spending less time working for the same employer, compounding the continuity of care issue and pushing the issue of coverage portability An increasing number of workers are also laboring under alternative arrangements such as part-time job relationships or independent contractor agreements.[81] These hard working and often entrepreneurial individuals are not captured by an employer-based system. Finally, the employer-based health insurance plans would do little to capture the 11.8 million individuals who are working in the United States illegally.

However, individual health care plans carry significant disadvantages as well. First, there are higher costs associated with their administration and sales, tending to drive up their premiums. Additionally, without the discipline of having money regularly allocated to the carrier, remission of a periodic premium can be inconsistent and its effects quite painful. The absence of risk averaging makes individual insurance premiums subject to wide fluctuations, and with the present legislative design, significant tax advantages exist for employer-based insurance plans.

If the playing field is legislatively leveled on accessibility, a shift towards greater participation in individual insurance plans can be expected, thus freeing the nation from its present dependence on employer-based health insurance.[79] The tax disadvantages most states impart on the individual insurance model can be modified to make this a more palatable option. Secondly, pseudo-group plans can be created to volume average the insurer's risk and help stabilize prices. Premium guarantees can be afforded to younger, healthier patients who sign on with an insurance company earlier in life while the probability of requiring expensive care is lower. In return, the insured's premium rate can be guaranteed later in life when he is more apt to incur higher health care expenses. Finally, removing preexisting-conditions-clauses would free the individual to transition to another plan as he sees fit.

Julio Gonzalez, M.D.

The Independent Health Coverage Council

Perhaps the most revolting and threatening example of government-intervention on health care is the Independent Health Coverage Council proposed in the Baucus Plan. This Council is a federal agency designed to regulate every aspect of the health care industry. It would be so intrusive as to be tasked with defining "coverage" and "affordability" and would play a major role in defining "high-quality" and "cost- effective care". The Council would also be responsible for providing appropriate oversight and collecting and maintaining pay-for-performance information. The powers of this agency to regulate the different aspects of the health care system would be all-pervasive, giving the government the ultimate ability to shape health care delivery in whatever direction it desires.

Examples abound within the Baucus Plan of how this massive regulation entitlement would play out. Perhaps the most elemental and deceiving of these is in the arena of health insurance premiums. Firstly, the Baucus Plan calls for the prohibition of premium adjustments related to risk. Additionally, any insurance company that participates in the Insurance Exchange must also subject itself to the scrutiny of government price regulation.

Three levels of insurance products that would vary with the level of coverage would be developed by the Independent Health Coverage Council and managed by the Health Insurance Exchange. The prices of these three products would be set so that they would remain within a specified price range.

The thought of government fixing prices for private industry is intimidating enough; however, an even greater assault on freedom and professional independence is launched under the guise of quality improvement and accountability. What makes this such an easy vehicle for manipulation is the desirability of the goal. Every responsible physician strives for it. Every patient demands it. Indeed, improving quality is an ongoing challenge for the medical industry.

However, when carriers get involved in the push for quality, ample room is created for these forces to promote agendas that are not always in line with the improvement of patient care. For example, when insurance companies speak of quality indicators, they are often really speaking of the financial efficacy with which their money is being spent. Of course, these two priorities are often complimentary. However, all too often, these two ways of judging outcomes -- health care quality and financial efficiency -- do not correlate. What the third party payer sells to the consumer as quality control (and Congress sells to its constituents) is actually cost containment, often carried out at the expense of quality.

One example of how these two priorities conflict is the "health care excellence" list. These are lists of physicians accumulated by an insurance company that rank or include physicians based on measures of physician outcomes. Physicians included in this list either receive a bonus or are placed on a list of preferred providers publishable to its enrollees. Unfortunately, the quality indicators are generally not designed by the providers and are not based on any scientifically approved methods. What's more, no attempt is made to correct the results of these indicators for the severity of the disease present in the patients encountered. The actual indicators and calculations are usually not published, and there is no requirement for an insurance company to do so. The result of these efforts could certainly be a valid attempt at producing a poorly designed list of quality physicians. Alternatively, such lists could merely serve as a way of rewarding those physicians who make the most profit for a particular carrier under the guise of quality.

The Center for Medicare and Medicaid Services has rolled out a number of programs designed to improve the "quality of care" provided by its participants. The first of these is a pay-for-reporting program disguised as a pay-for-performance program issued by Medicare. In it, physicians are asked to report their compliance with 16 quality indicators that CMS has designated as desirable. These range from placing a congestive heart failure patient on a specific type of blood pressure medication to an orthopaedic surgeon counseling a fracture patient about bone quality and osteoporosis. In an obvious attempt by administrators and non-physicians to manipulate health care in ways they were not trained, a small bonus is provided at the end of the year to those who comply. This program and others like it ignore the fact that not every treatment, even the most innocuous ones, is beneficial to every patient. For example, greater than 60 percent of patients covered by Medicare have more than one chronic medical condition. In some of these cases, the administration of specific kinds of blood pressure medications is contraindicated. As a result, the physician will not administer the medication (hopefully) despite the financial pressure to do so. The result of providing the patient with the higher quality treatment, then, is to lower the physician's compliance percentage and place him closer to not qualifying for the added bonus.

Another flawed method is the surgical report card. In the 1990s, certain insurance companies issued report cards for cardiothoracic surgeons based on surgical outcomes. The logic was that if the physician scored better than a certain minimum number, he would be rewarded with a bonus payment. The result was to induce the very same "cherry-picking" strategies that Senator Baucus alluded to in his objections to physician ownership of hospitals. Many surgeons and health care institutions decided they were better off taking care of the simpler, less-involved patients in exchange for improved outcomes scores. As a result, sicker patients were finding it increasingly difficult to receive care, and overall access to care suffered.

The same effect can be predicted for the Medicare quality reporting program. Physicians will realize that it pays to see the simpler patient rather than tackling the more difficult ones who will demand more time and effort.

The same potentially deleterious effects can also be expected from the "never events" program instituted by CMS in October, 2008, in accordance with the

Deficit Reduction Act of 2005. In this program, CMS reserves the right to deny payment to a hospital for the additional costs of treating a condition resulting from a never-event. Examples of these never-events include "hospital acquired" methicillin resistant Staphylococcus aureus (MRSA) infections, wound infections, retained instruments, pressure ulcers, and deep venous thromboses. According to CMS, these events are so egregious that they represent a serious deficiency in health care delivery and should not be reimbursed.

This approach defies any attempt at logic or scientific merit. Firstly, many of the conditions listed are not universally preventable, and their acquisition does not necessarily indicate a quality breach on the part of the hospital or care provider. For example, we know that despite adequate anticoagulation with warfarin, aspirin, or low-molecular-weight heparin products, about 12 percent of patients who have undergone lower-extremity joint reconstructions will develop a deep venous thrombosis, and anywhere between one in 2,000 and one in 5,000 will have a lethal embolus. Again, this is despite all appropriate countermeasures. Yet, in the eyes of CMS, the development of a thromboembolism following a joint reconstructive procedure or spine surgery is listed as a never event.

Another example is MRSA infection. Medicare has said that if a patient develops an MRSA infection in the hospital, it will be deemed as hospital acquired, and Medicare will not pay for services relating to the treatment of this condition. The problem is that the presumption of an MRSA infection being hospital acquired is no longer valid. The striking evidence of this lies in the numerous cases of MRSA infections and even deaths in patients having no recent contact with a hospital or patient. In my hospital, for example, the emergency room physicians have started treating patients with community-acquired, spider-bite-related skin infections with sulfamethoxazole, instead of the cephalosporin antibiotic they used to prescribe. Why? Because of the increased incidence of patients presenting with community-acquired MRSA infections. Indeed, the only effect this never event measure is having is to increase the level of defensive medicine, a new phenomenon in health care I call "fiscally defensive medicine", and a direct result of the implementation of ill-conceived quality control measures by third party payers. In order to help defend themselves against a Medicare accusation of hospital-acquired infection, many centers are performing screening cultures for MRSA for either a subsegment of patients or all patients either admitted or due to be admitted to the hospital. In so doing they hope to identify the patients who are carrying MRSA in their skin at the time of, or prior to, the admission so that the hospital may protect its reimbursement. By and large, the results of these tests will have no effect in the treatment rendered, but they are being done as part of this new wave of fiscally defensive medicine. The net effect is to increase health care treatment costs without any benefits to patient care. In essence, by meddling in issues of health care administration, proponents of quality reviews are essentially causing the very effect they are trying to avoid -- that of increasing health care costs and decreasing the fiscal efficiency of delivery.

These examples help to describe the deleterious effects many of these well-intentioned programs are having on health care providers and patients alike. It would stand to reason that jurisdictional authorities would do everything in their power from discouraging providers and health care institutions from treating more complicated patients. However, many of the programs proposed in the Baucus Plan do just that.

One example is the proposition of reimbursing admissions taking place within 30 days of a previous admission at half the usual reimbursement rate. If there were even a single physician in the Senate Finance Committee, or if Senator Baucus had sought any insight from a practicing physician, he would have known how much physicians and hospitals detest "bounce-backs". Readmissions are the source of great stress for physicians because of the administrative hassles associated with these repeat admissions, the labor-intensive nature of these events, and more importantly, the fact that a bounce-back represents a patient whose clinical problem has not been solved or stabilized.

Nothing is detested more by a physician than an unsolved medical problem. It is not only the source of a great workload, but it is also the cause of great dismay and emotional distress. Nobody seeks a readmission as a source of revenue or compensation, and it is something that all parties involved are actively trying to prevent. It is therefore not worth trying to discourage, because physicians and institutions alike are already working hard to try to avoid these events. As such, threatening to pay half rates for readmissions will only achieve one aim: to discourage physicians from taking care of the more complicated patients because these are the ones who are more apt to be readmitted.

Another example of a proposed plan with a questionable return is the pay-for-performance plan. In pay-for-performance strategies, the carrier will match cost savings from treatments of certain medical conditions with physician reimbursement. Essentially, if the provider organization can demonstrate a cost savings to the carrier, the clinician group will then be allowed to keep a portion of the savings. It is hoped that in so doing, the clinician will be motivated to cost contain and effect a reduction in total health care costs.

A number of pay-for-performance demonstrations have been implemented by Medicare.[82] In one example, a physician group practice treating patients with congestive heart failure is challenged with developing innovative ways of detecting the condition earlier in its course so as to prevent expensive admissions. In one demonstration, the group developed a strategy whereby patients would be called at home and asked for their weights. Any patient with rapid weight gain, a sign of fluid retention and worsening heart failure, would then be treated as an outpatient before the problem spiraled out of control. It is estimated that in the five-months after establishing this practice, the clinic avoided 65 hospital admissions at a cost savings of $500,000. [82] Potentially, the clinicians stood to take some of that money home. However, according to the participants involved in the demonstration, the approach was labor-intensive, requiring multiple individuals to be involved in the process of patient identification and follow-through, using resources not available to the majority of health care providers in this country.

Dr. Doug Carr of the Billings Clinic, a participant in the demonstration study, noted that if all the cost-savings interventions were implemented, the team would be able to save approximately $9.5 million. As a result, the clinic would stand to make about $3.5 million for their success. According Dr. Carr, the practice would have spent approximately $4 million in the effort, causing them to work at a net loss of $500,000 for their participation in the program. And this is for a physician group practice with scores of employees at their command and millions of dollars at their disposal.

Tied into the concept of coordinated care and value based payments is physician group practices (PGP). The concept behind these entities is that health care should not be administered by a single individual. Instead, health care, especially care for individuals with chronic conditions, should be managed by a multi-specialty group. When a patient enrolls in a practice, or becomes one of its patients, he will be treated by a coordinated compendium of resources that include generalists (non-specialist physicians such as internists and family practice physicians), specialists, dietitians, physiatrists, etc. The patient would then move easily between specialties inside the practice walls to receive a coordinated health care approach that would concentrate on health maintenance and preventive methods. The result would be that everyone would be attached to a large, coordinated practice that would track patient health indicators and intervene at appropriate times.

This model is certainly attractive, in theory. However, what will suffer from such an approach is the bastion of personal medical care as we know it today… the solo physician. A multitude of studies demonstrate that patients value a continued relationship with their physicians.[83,84] The establishment and protection of an ongoing, confidential, and personal relationship between physician and patient has been pivotal to the philosophy of medical practice in this country. Physicians and patients alike want to know they have someone they can turn to when they get sick or need medical care. Patients want to know that they have someone whom they can trust, with whom they have a positive, personal relationship, and who is familiar with their health care needs. Physicians value the opportunity to continue with someone's care plan without intervention from competing opinions or interruptions in the overall plan for that particular patient's health. They also find the familiarity with the patient's personality, expectations and medical history invaluable in their ability to provide reliable and dependable medical care.

The physician group practice model is a direct threat to that concept. The group practice model assumes that one can substitute one physician for another. It also implies that although one institution may be responsible for the patient's care, no one person is. The market manipulations and incentives instituted by the Baucus Plan will be such that the private, independent physician will eventually be phased out, not because the model is so expensive or inefficient, but rather because the government decided that this model is not the one it preferred. In the end medical practices will have to respond, not to market pressures placed on them by patient preferences and consumer demands, but by government engineered financial choke holds that may not reflect the desires of the American consumer.

Since these PGPs are built on the back of

generalists, the Baucus Plan will aim at increasing the number of general medicine physicians in the workforce. It argues that because reimbursement practices tend to favor specialty physicians, the present health care system is skewed towards specialty medicine and away from general, all-encompassing care. This view of medicine and the relationship between specialty and generalist physicians is completely misguided. Health care is becoming more specialty- oriented simply because the intricacies of our understanding of the human body is becoming increasingly complex, as are the interventions available. What would have been learned by a student decades ago about an organ system in a year or two now has become so complex and intricate that it may take decades to master, or perhaps necessitate splitting into subspecialties. The other and more important reason for the trend toward specialization in medicine is quite simple: patients are demanding it. And because they are participants in the greatest and most complex health care system in the world they are able to get it.

The fact that some specialty physicians are paid more than generalists can be traced to two very simple reasons that are completely unrelated to any skewing of the market: 1) there are fewer specialists practicing within each field; and 2) they take longer to produce. In fact, as anyone who has gone through medical training knows, there is a great disincentive to pursuing specialty training: time, usually between two to five extra years of youthful life. This disincentive is what prevents more candidates from pursuing specialty training. It takes great time, effort, and sacrifice to achieve that extra degree of training at a point in one's life where friends in other fields and many colleagues are building wealth and raising children. The extra but insufficient compensation for these people is designed to make up for that sacrifice. It is specifically not due to an overvaluation of specialty care. Negative governmental policies designed to dissuade physician candidates from pursuing specialty training will only serve to compound the problem of access to care. It behooves health policy experts, therefore, to protect the interests of both specialty and generalist physicians by letting the consumer demand how much the relative demands of these services should be, not government policy.

Additionally, as opposed to the implications made in "Call to Action," there are countless patients who are better treated by having the specialist serve as their medical home instead of the generalist. An example of this may be the patient with labile diabetes whose care may best be managed by an endocrinology specialist.

Adding to the erroneous presumptions of Senator Baucus' view of medicine is the thought that having a patient treated by a generalist helps to save health care dollars. The misuse of MRIs serves as a perfect example of the misconceptions behind this position. According to analysts, the price of unnecessary MRI scans may be costing consumers $30 billion.[85] One source of this unnecessary spending is the misplaced practice of generalists ordering MRIs for patients they are preparing to refer to a specialist when the specialist does not need the study.[86] In this case, as well as countless others, early referral to a specialist would actually save the carrier and the consumer money and time by avoiding unnecessary testing.

Due to the incredible complexity of the health

care system and health care delivery, well-meaning interventions designed to improve quality may actually end up diminishing it. The fact is that there are only two ways one can truly assess quality in health care delivery. The first is to have outcome markers implemented with premorbid health quality evaluations and corrections made for the health population studied. This randomly assigned, anonymously reported information would then be analyzed by a statistician for outcome scores corrected for the disease severity. A performance index could then be assigned to each practitioner and their outcomes better compared. Doing this would be prohibitively expensive, nullifying any attempt at cost containment. Another way of assessing quality would be to have an impartial, specialty-trained physician audit a number of cases, observe the target physician practice, and interview a number of the physician's patients to get an idea of the quality of care being delivered. Again, such an undertaking would be impossible to perform in an economically viable manner due to the sheer intensity of such a program.

I would therefore propose that third party payers and the government abandon these misguided, unfairly applied, counterproductive quality initiatives and allow the health care providers, the civil justice system, and the market regulate the health care system. Once again, policymakers need to accept that they possess neither the insight nor the resources necessary to intelligently apply these interventions without risking damaging the system.[87] The best approach is to trust the system that produces the physicians, and let doctors do the doctoring and their own surveillance.

CHAPTER 7:

EFFECTS ON THE WORKFORCE

What are the effects of these changes on the people providing care? The answer to this question is the crux behind the concerns over the present health care reform movement. Previously in this volume we explored the aging nature of our health care providers and how an increasing number of them were in a position to consider early retirement or reducing the number of patients they see. The compendium of conditions that would lead to a mass exodus of actively practicing physicians in this country is rapidly materializing. Key to these conditions are issues of reimbursement, excessive administrative oversight, and litigious risk.

The Medicaid system provides us with examples of the factors afflicting the health care system in this regard. Despite the matching funds allocated by the federal government, many states still offer less than Medicare reimbursement for health care provider services. As a result, Medicaid patients have few options related to where and from whom they receive their care. The Center for Studying Health System Change has found decreasing physician participation in Medicaid programs nationwide, forcing patients to gravitate to large centers, hospitals, and teaching institutions to receive their care.[88] Central to this trend is the poor compensation (69 percent of Medicare reimbursement rates on the average[89]) and increased administrative load associated with dealing with this insurance plan. In some states such as Texas, the fraction of physicians not accepting new Medicaid insurance patients is about 60 percent.[90]

These issues are also threatening provider participation in Medicare. In a survey of 8,955 physicians conducted in 2007, 64 percent of physicians reported that they would stop accepting new Medicare patients if the 21 percent cut in reimbursement scheduled to take place in 2010 were to go into effect.[91] Medicare Advantage plans, the privately managed Medicare insurances, are plagued with similar restrictions stemming from the administrative burdens these plans place on physicians and resentment over carriers being paid approximately 112 percent of Medicare reimbursement fees for physician services while they only pay physicians the standard 100 percent Medicare allotted rate.

In the state of Florida, the Department of Health has released its first annual physician workforce report assembled from the results of a mandatory questionnaire linked to physician relicensure.[92] Thirteen percent of physicians in Florida said they would reduce or discontinue their practice over the next five years. Only 31 percent said they were taking emergency room call or worked in an emergency room, with an additional 11 percent stating that they would reduce their involvement with emergency room care. Eighteen percent of radiologists said they were going to reduce or discontinue reading mammograms. Only 40 percent of physicians identifying themselves as providing obstetrical care actually delivered babies, and another 14 percent said they would discontinue providing obstetrical services over the next two years.[93]

And the situation stands to get worse. Not only is there a significant number of physicians looking at exiting the field or reducing their involvement in it, there also seems to be a shortage of young physicians to pick up the slack. According to the Florida Department of Health workforce report, only 36 percent of physicians practicing in Florida are 45 years old or younger.[93] This correlates with the information reported earlier in this text about the nationwide workforce statistics.

The overall implication this data suggests the physician workforce will weaken over time. This is a trend that has not been seen in this country since its inception and correlates with the increasing intrusions of government and administrators in the practice of medicine. Evidence in support of this direct correlation can be gathered from the 2008 Florida Department of Health physician's workforce report in which 63.85 percent of physicians cited the top reasons for changing, reducing, or discontinuing their practice as being ones under the direct control of politicians, bureaucrats, and administrators (liability - 27.38 percent, reimbursement - 24.36 percent, and regulatory and administrative burden -12.11 percent).[94]

The quintessential concern for the American public regarding health care reform should be the destructive effect these measures of manipulation are having on the most important element of the health care system: the people who provide the care. Instead of improving the environment in which they practice and incentivizing them to remain engaged in health care, we are chasing them away with reimbursement cuts that are unparalleled in any other sector of the American economy, increased litigious risks, and an increasingly onerous administrative burden. And what's worse, the word is getting out to our nation's youngsters about the diminishing returns and the increasing burdens associated with becoming a health care provider causing them to consider applying their skills elsewhere.

As this trend progresses, this country will have to increasingly rely on inferior applicants and foreign medical graduates to supply a greater portion of our care, a tendency that can already be documented. We have already noted how the United States has been importing physicians from other countries (this figure is presently about 25 percent and rising). In Europe, the model of the administrative hassles and logistic inefficiencies that our health care reformers insist on emulating, higher concentrations of foreign physicians abound.* Following this model will result in a progressive loss of control over the quality of medicine in this country and on an increased reliance on foreign countries for the maintenance of the American health care workforce.

---

* In the England, the European country with the highest number of foreign medical graduates about 47.5 percent of its workforce is comprised of foreign physicians. The percentage for Ireland is 30.94 percent, for Malta 23.1 percent.[95]

CHAPTER 8:

THE COST OF HEALTH CARE

Where Is Our Money Going?

At 2.1 trillion dollars per year, the United States spends exorbitantly more on health care than any other country in the world. This discrepancy remains regardless of whether the amount is analyzed as a percentage of GDP or a per capita rate expenditure. One explanation of the discrepancy may be that, as the richest nation in the world, the United States is apt to spend more on its health care system than other countries. Although there is a general correlation between a country's per capita health expenditure and its GDP, the amount that Americans spend on health care vastly exceeds that predicted by this ratio.[96] According to the McKinsey Global Institute, an organization that studies global economic policy and expenditure patterns, the discrepancy between what the United States spends on its health care and the amount that would be expected based on its per capita GDP is $650 billion.[96] The question is, why?

The CMS National Health Expenditure Accounts Data for 2006 provides some information insight into this issue. Figure 8.1 summarizes the breakdown of heath care expenditures for 2006. According to this data, 52% of the nation's health care costs are allocated to hospital care, and physician and clinical services.

Julio Gonzalez, M.D.

Seven percent is allocated to administrative costs. The second largest expenditure goes to the "other spending" category, which includes services performed by non-physician professionals, home health care, durable medical equipment, over-the-counter medications and sundries, research, structures and equipment. Of note, is that according to this data, administrative and net costs only accounted for about 7% of the money spent on health care. Although administrative costs in the United States can be reduced, it certainly does not seem to account for an overwhelming percentage of health care costs.

Neither does the expense for providing for our aging population. Figure 8.2 compares the amount the United States spends on health care per capita as in each age group. The seemingly exponential increase in health care spending with increasing age would tempt one to conclude that total health care spending for the higher age groups would be enormous. However, Figure 8.3, which looks at the total health care spending within those groups, demonstrates that this is indeed not the case.

There is other evidence to dispel this myth. In Table 4.2 we see that neither the average population age of a country, its life expectancy, or the percent of inhabitants that are older than 64 is dramatically different in the United States from that of any of the countries we are using as benchmarks. Additionally, although our population is increasing in age, this number changes at a very slow rate, certainly slower than the rate at which the expenses of our health care system is increasing.[97]

Health care provider reimbursement is also commonly blamed for high health care costs. Our recent review of the history of physician reimbursement in Chapter 2 argues otherwise. What's more, if one considers the amount of money required for health care to compete with other fields that recruit from the highest tiers of educational development and accomplishment, one immediately realizes that physicians are amongst the most *underpaid* group of professionals in this country.[98]

After its extensive investigations into the matter, the McKinsey Global Institute has provided some explanations to account for the high and ever-increasing costs of health care in the United States. Amongst these are 1) provider capacity growth in response to high outpatient margins, 2) the judgment based nature of physician care, 3) technological innovation that drives prices up, 4) demand growth that appears to be due to greater availability of supply and 5) relative price-insensitive patients with limited out-of-pocket expenses.[99]

Of course, one would expect these different factors to have varying influences on the upward trend of health care costs in the United States. For example, the judgment-based nature of medicine should have equal weight in influencing total health care expenditures regardless of the country involved as this factor represents a truism of medical practice that transcends borders. However, how aggressively a society questions the judgment of a physician (the legal environment in which the physician finds himself) will play a significant role in the practice patterns displayed by its providers and its associated costs. Technological innovation is also a global influence, but one that is tempered by a particular region's ability to access such innovations (cost sensitivity)*. Although the second factor is somewhat influenced by legislative pressures, in a free-market system the first, third and fourth factors are all under the direct influence of the market pressures--i.e. the fifth factor, or price insensitivity.

The importance of price-insensitivity on inflating the costs of health care is repeatedly demonstrated by our historical experience. In Chapter 2, we reviewed how the appearance of Medicare in 1965 may have been single-handedly responsible for 40% of the increase in the per capita spending that took place over the ensuing 35 years.[28] But this is not the only example. Most recently our country has experienced a dramatic increase in pharmaceutical spending largely in response to the establishment of the Medicare pharmaceutical coverage plan or Medicare Part D.[100] The high volume of unnecessary provider visits with which our country's military health care system wrestles serves as further testimony to this relationship (Chapter 2).

As such, any serious attempt at reforming health care with the aim of cutting down on its total expenditures must account for the inverse relationship between the consumer's financial stake in the health care provided and overall spending. It is interesting that the Baucus Plan, President Obama's vision for health care reform, the Democrat party model for health care reform, and indeed

* I say cost-sensitivity as opposed to price-sensitivity in this case since the influence on a region's access to specific technologies revolves around the cost of supplying the product to its population. Price-sensitivity as used in this text is the awareness of the amount of money a consumer has to pay within a certain network for a product or service compared to the price of the same or similar product or service provided by a competing network.

126

the modern health care reform movement all ignore this basic tenet and move to even further divorce the individual from his responsibility for the cost of his care. Senator Baucus has already conceded that the implementation of universal coverage will cost this country approximately 100-150 billion dollars. If history serves us correctly, such a plan would cost us even more as the consumer, increasingly shielded from the costs of his care and aware that addressing his issues is the responsibility of someone other than himself, will seek consultation for problems that he may have otherwise felt did not merit formal intervention. More significantly, the fiscally protected patient will demand full evaluation of his health problems, particularly if less involved evaluations demonstrate the absence of serious disease without the identification of a specific diagnosis.

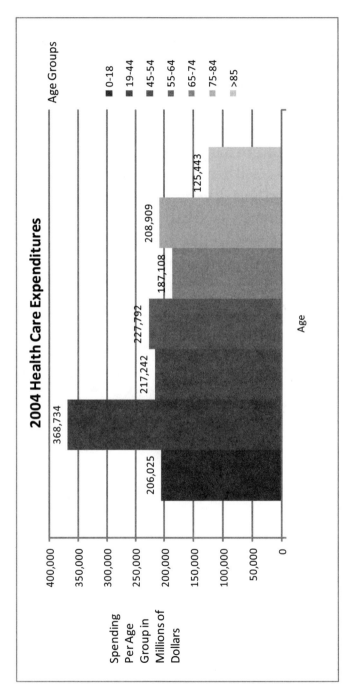

Figure 8.1 - U.S. Health Care Expenditures by age group

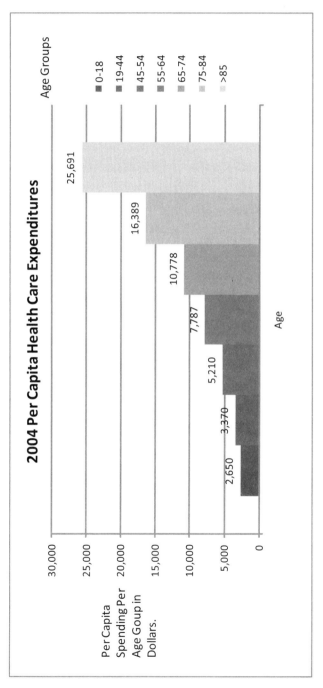

Figure 8.2 - U.S. Health Care Expenditures per capita within age groups

The Nation's Health Dollar
Calendar Year 2006: Where It Went

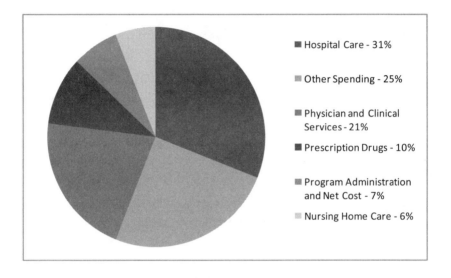

Legend:
- Hospital Care - 31%
- Other Spending - 25%
- Physician and Clinical Services - 21%
- Prescription Drugs - 10%
- Program Administration and Net Cost - 7%
- Nursing Home Care - 6%

NOTE: Other spending includes dental services, other professional services, home health, durable medical products, over-the-counter medicines and sundries, public health, other personal health care, research and structures and equipment.

SOURCE: Centers for Medicare and Medicaid Services, Office of the Actuary, National Health Statistics Group

Figure 8.3-Breakdown of the Nation's Health Care Dollars Allocation in 2006.

What Are We Buying?

Although price insensitivity has been posited as the driving force behind our country's relative high health care expenditures, another factor has correlated strongly with high national health care costs. As mentioned previously, a 2001 analysis demonstrated a linear relationship between national per capita GDP health care costs and performance in the WHO's responsiveness index.[17] Although the WHO's assessment of national health care systems was published in 2000, it remains the most recent and complete assessment of the relative responsiveness of national health care systems throughout the globe. It would therefore be interesting to note whether this correlation still holds up using the latest per capita GDP expenditure figures.

Figure 8.4 demonstrates the relationship between the WHO responsiveness indices published in 2000 and the 2006 developed countries' per capita GDP health care expenditures. Evaluation of this data shows preservation of the linear relationship between total health care dollars spent and system responsiveness.

It is therefore clear that what the American people are paying for and are all too willing to fund is the same thing that they pay for in any other industry: responsiveness. Whether they are dealing with consumer products, professional services or health care, Americans, in their staunch independence and unyielding demand for quality and service have driven their health care system to become the most responsive in the world. This then, is the underlying conflict between that changes policymakers are trying to forcibly effect and what the American public wants. It is the underlying fact that drives Secretary Designee of the Department of Health and Humans Services, Mr. Thomas Daschle, to call doctors and patients losers in his plans to reform health care. Through the government's concerted efforts at cutting total health care costs and by the relinquishing control of our health care system to the government, what we are essentially sacrificing is this system's ability to respond to *our*, demands, not that of the government. It stands to reason therefore that Americans will never be satisfied with the autocratic changes being implemented upon the American health care system by government reformers.

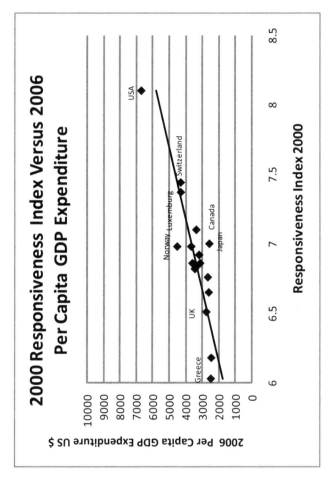

Figure 8.4- Relationship Between Responsiveness and Per Capita GDP

Julio Gonzalez, M.D.

The Fallacy of Preventive Medicine As a Cost-Containment Measure

> *Preventive medicine: Interventions designed to avert and avoid disease. The branch of medicine concerned with preventing disease. A branch of medicine dealing with methods of preventing disease.*

The benefits of preventive medicine in the improvement of lifestyle, prolonging productivity and fostering feelings of self-worth are indisputable. Individuals who make healthy lifestyle choices such as avoiding smoking, maintaining ideal body weight, lowering cholesterol and participating in a regular exercise program score better in health assessments than their less engaged counterparts. Indeed, as a rule, these individuals have fewer hospitalizations, fewer physician contacts and are able to keep disease processes from progressing for longer periods of time. It is therefore tempting to say that engaging a population in an aggressive preventive medicine program will lower the costs associated with health care. Indeed the temptation is so great that The Baucus Plan even includes provisions for improving neighborhoods as part of its preventive medicine program.[101]

The thought of a government run health care system becoming responsible for the promotion of "healthier communities" is of course, absurd, and counter to the perception of the role of the American government. But there it is logically espoused as an extension of government's newly assumed role for health maintenance and disease prevention. It certainly would not be too far-fetched to envision the argument of removing guns from neighborhoods despite the provisions of the second amendment. This step, of course, would be closely followed by one that regulates the types of foods and beverages sold within a community or perhaps to certain individuals of the community, all in the name of the government's role as health czar. The scenarios seem preposterous, but if legislators can defend the government's role in community improvement on the basis of health promotion, then these other measures cannot be too far behind.

Not only is the thought of government having an expansive role in the promotion of disease prevention potentially ominous, but there are many studies indicating that such an approach could do very little to lower the overall costs of health care to a population.[102,103] There are a number of problems with preventive medicine as a cost containment strategy. For starters, not all interventions are cost effective. For example, it appears that the administration of flu vaccines is a cost-effective step for preventing disease-related expenditures. However, screening all elderly patients for hypertension would probably not meet with the same cost-containment goals. Additionally, cost containment strategies in one group may not be beneficial for another. Smoking cessation serves as a perfect example of just such a situation. Whereas smoking cessation instituted in the third decade of life carries innumerable benefits to patient and society alike, demanding this measure from a 90 year old from a preventive medicine standpoint is certainly suspect. The thought sounds amazingly obvious, but the number of extreme-old-age patients who are presently treated with cholesterol lowering drugs and blood thinners baffles the imagination, especially when one considers that its benefits for that age group in preventing anything other cost containment efforts is doubtful.

One must also bear in mind that many of the efforts touted as "preventive" in nature are ones that represent active treatment of a disease with the intent of keeping its sequelae in check. Preventing admissions to a hospital from complications of a disease is not preventive medicine. This is merely an appropriate approach for the treatment of an underlying condition. It may be cost effective and help keep people out of the hospital, but it hardly qualifies as preventive medicine. For example, treating patients who have HIV with antiretroviral medications in an effort to keep them from developing AIDS is not preventive medicine. However, abstinence, monogamy and the use of appropriate barrier contraception to keep one from contracting HIV is.

Another reason that preventive medicine may not be as helpful as its proponents tout it to be is that many of the people targeted with these measure are amongst the healthiest of the population and not the biggest consumers of health care at all.

There is also the issue of future cost increases as a result of preventive medicine. As we have seen, the per capita costs of health care increases exponentially with advancing age (See Table 8.1). A sound, carefully orchestrated preventive medicine program can help prolong life and improve quality of life for some time, but the body will inevitably fail. As a result, diminishing the incidence of one disease will only serve to substitute it for the life-ending process of another. For example, the rate of lung cancer as a cause of death amongst men has diminished in response to our country's smoking cessation efforts, but these are being traded for the higher number of deaths from other cancers and dementia. Similarly, in women, we have seen the number of deaths from cervical cancer diminish over the past forty years, its influence only to be traded for an increasing prevalence of breast cancer. During the present decade, thanks to early detection efforts and improved treatments, both the incidence of and mortality from breast cancer has diminished. But these will only be displaced by a higher incidence of another illness that affects those who avoided getting the disease, such as other types of cancer, heart disease, stroke or dementia. The unreported irony is that the country's success at controlling one disease is the very reason that allows the incidence of others to climb. One can therefore conclude that from a health economics standpoint preventive medicine may serve more as a cost delayer than a cost constrainer. This attestation lends credence to the words of Dr. Robert Evans who was quoted as saying, "the cheapest approach is to have your coronary at 62 and go."[102]

Julio Gonzalez, M.D.

End of Life Care.

Another area where health care costs can be better controlled is at the end of life. It is estimated that 27% of Medicare's yearly budget, approximately $327 billion dollars, is spent to care for patients in their final year of life.[104] How much of that was spent on heroic, futile efforts at effecting cures for patients with limited hopes of survival is certainly worthy of study. Redirecting those funds towards efforts revolving around supportive management would likely result in a significant reduction in health care spending and represent a more appropriate mode of resource allocation, not to mention being more humane on the patient and loved ones.

CHAPTER 9:

CONCLUSIONS

Despite the affirmations from proponents for modern health care reform, the United States has the most intricate, technologically advanced, sophisticated health care system in the world and is doing a much better job at providing health care for a larger and more diverse group of people than any other country. It is a system that was built from individuality, resourcefulness, opportunity and innovation. Like the country that houses it, the American health care system serves as a beacon of technological development emulated the world over, this despite the presence of a taxing strain from an illegal, largely uninsured, immigrant population that is 11.8 million people strong.

Efforts at discrediting the American health care system are often based on unsubstantiated information and mischaracterized representations of epidemiological and demographic data. Chief amongst these are the infant mortality rate and data regarding the number of uninsured residing in this country. It is crucial therefore, that these numbers be appropriately defined without hyperbole or exaggerations so that a true attempt at problem identification can be made which can then be followed by a more effective corrective strategy. For example, the often-cited number of uninsured in this country of 46 million individuals includes many groups for whom the American taxpayer is not motivated to assist in the procurement of health care coverage. These inhabitants include the illegal immigrant population and individuals from higher income brackets who can afford health care insurance but have opted against purchasing it. After adjusting for the influence of these two groups, the number of uninsured for which a significant proportion of the American people would consider assisting is no more than 16.3 million. Additionally, the relationship between disparities in health indicators and the absence of insurance coverage may not be a function of insurance status but to the influence of poverty. Identifying the root cause of these disparities prior to effecting any corrections is crucial as it would help prevent the implementation of ineffective corrections upon the health care system that end up weakening rather than strengthening it.

Despite the absolute marvel that is American health care, there are significant shortcomings that leave room for improvement. The exceedingly high degree of health care expenditure, amounting to 2.1 trillion dollars, or 16% of the GDP is one example. Another is the presence of health care disparities between socioeconomic and ethnic groups. The magnitude and the extent of these problems and the degree to which a concerted effort should be made towards their amelioration are matters of great debate.

The Baucus Plan as described in Senator Max Baucus's (D-MT) white paper on health care reform called "Call to Action Health Care Reform 2009" provides a succinct summary of what modern health care reform proponents envision as possible solutions to the problems affecting our health care system. It provides great insight into the mind set of the leaders of the modern health care reform movement. The underlying philosophy of the

Plan is that greater government involvement is needed in order to address the two major shortcomings of the American health care system: excess costs and a lack of universality of health care coverage.

In its zeal to embrace universal health care coverage and tighter government scrutiny, the Baucus Plan ignores many of the even greater shortcomings experienced in the health care models from which it seeks to borrow. Chief amongst these are the severe restrictions in health care independence and the poor responsiveness (long wait times for treatment) inherent to these systems. It wrongly assumes that such restrictions will be well tolerated in our country. Additionally, the Baucus Plan holds that the government, with all of its resources and experts, has the insight necessary to accurately predict the consequences of their manipulations on the health care field and its markets. One large problem inherent to the formulation of the plan is the exclusion of stakeholders in the health care reform process, most likely because Senator Baucus and the generators of "Call to Action" know that the vast majority of rank-and-file health care providers will be opposed to the stipulations inherent to the Plan.

Also dispelled as a temporary investment is the $100 $150 billion start-up costs necessary to initiate a universal health care coverage plan. Once again, the Baucus Plan assumes that through tighter regulation, the government will be able to make up for this loss. However, there appears to be no substance to this belief. For one, the thought that the government can provide health care with a far lower overhead than private carriers is misplaced. Additionally, the presumption that government intervention can help result in lowering total health care expenditures ignores the recurrent and predictable pattern of increasing health care spending associated with greater government involvement.

Perhaps the most devastating effect of these changes will be on the strength of our health care workforce, a resilient, underpaid and stubbornly independent group of individuals who are well aware of their respective expertise in their fields. Any attempt at increasing regulation and expanding the administrative burden with which they must function tips them closer to seeking early retirement or reducing their participation in the system. A mass exodus of these physicians and health care providers will not be tolerated by the health care system, especially in the face of the emerging "baby boomer tidal wave" and will lead to critical understaffing challenges, if not the downright collapse of the system. Adding to this element is the increasing difficulty in recruitment of young, bright, American-trained individuals to fill in the gaps developed by the expanded attrition that such excess regulation and micromanagement will cause.

Another presumption that appears to be in error is the concept upholding that an increasing role of the employer in funding and administering the non-Medicare health care system is a viable avenue to pursue. The predictable, negative effects on economic growth, mean earned wages, unemployment and poverty levels seem to be ignored. There are also numerous disadvantages to an employer-based system, including portability constraints, lack of choices in selecting an appropriate health care plan to suit one's individual needs and a lack of individual accountability for one's health care. Additionally, the concept that the government and the employer should share in the responsibility of arranging for the country's health care flies directly in the face of the concept invoked in "Call to Action", namely, that arranging for health care coverage should be the responsibility of the individual. Such insulation of the individual from true responsibility for health and health care coverage as outlined in the Baucus Plan leads to the inference that the only responsibility placed by the Plan upon the individual is a legal one, meaning that anyone who does not get health care coverage under the Baucus Plan will be subject to legal repercussions such as fines and incarceration.

History has shown that in matters as complex and intricate as health care, no single entity is able to manipulate the system with reliably predictable results. In health care, as in any other multifaceted system the best way to proceed is to let the market take its course and let the individuals decide the form they desire their system to take. Such an approach is doomed to failure, however, if the individuals dictating the direction of the market are divorced from the consequences of their selections.

As is discussed in the upcoming chapter, an effort at true health care reform would be one that allows the stakeholders to take control of their product, lets the consumer negotiate their prices with their providers and actively encourages the most gifted minds of each generation to take up the life-long charge of caring for others.

CHAPTER 10:

RECOMMENDATIONS

Throughout this treatise, we have explored the strengths and weaknesses of the American health care system. We have analyzed the misconceptions and miscategorizations of its problems by the proponents of health care reform. As noted previously, the proposed changes to our health care system that are presently in the forefront of the minds of policy-makers and legislators, if enacted, will eventually serve to increase consumer dissatisfaction, stymie the drive for excellence ingrained in the health care workforce, diminish recruitment capabilities for future generations and perhaps have the unintended consequence of actually increasing health care costs. However, to provide criticisms of a plan without offering alternative solutions would represent an incomplete effort. Consequently, in this section, alternative approaches are offered for consideration. Some are very specific measures designed to address the identified concerns, others are merely provided as advice over how to approach the problem-solving process irrespective of which solution is selected.

Julio Gonzalez, M.D.

Give the Task of Health Care Reform to the Stakeholders

The first and most important recommendation is to allow the health care professionals to assume the role of reformers. The task of considering health care reform should be assigned to interested health care providers. It seems audacious for physicians, chiropractors and physical therapists to set out to reform the nation's judicial system. It is equally absurd to have lawyers and foreign policy experts redesign our health care system. If anything, a group of physicians, nurses, chiropractors, therapists and hospital administrators should be setting the agenda on health care reform with lawyers, economists and social policy experts serving as their advisors. As of this writing, there are twelve physicians in Congress. It makes absolutely no sense for the legislature to not employ the talents of these individuals in the endeavor of reforming our health care system. Committees charged with considering solutions to our health challenges should also seek the advice of practicing health care providers and encourage the offering of their ideas for consideration. It is likely the solutions proposed will be practical ones that stand a better chance of addressing real problems that are encountered in the day-to-day care of patients

Define the Problem

It is not sufficient to say that there are disparities in health care delivery and that the country is presently spending too much on health care. These are overall general realities that result from a series of shortcomings present in our society. The root causes of these shortcomings must be identified and defined. The solutions developed must address these specific shortcomings and not take the form of sweeping reforms that are hoped to correct the perceived problems while undercutting the system's strengths.

A number of specific examples of errors being presently made in this regard have already been discussed. These include confusing uninsured inhabitants with uninsured Americans, stating that we do not have universal access to health care, allowing flawed international statistics on health care delivery to be given weights that they do not deserve (the infant mortality rate, the WHO ranking scheme, etc) and confusing problems arising from lifestyle choices and poverty with problems arising from health care delivery.

Julio Gonzalez, M.D.

At First Do No Harm

This sacred adage of medical treatment will serve medical policymakers as well. The development of the American health care system with its intricacies and allure for innovation and change represents a miracle every bit as remarkable as the events that transpired in Philadelphia in 1776. The system that our country has enacted is one that allows for the delivery of a sophisticated and intricate product while promoting vehicles for change, ingenuity, and innovation. We *really* do not want to do *anything* to weaken this system or harm it in any way. In approaching any effort at reforming our methods of health care delivery we must constantly ask ourselves what is working now and preserve those successful elements. These elements have included a reliance on free-market principles with implemented checks designed to improve conditions for the poor and underserved. This overall framework has served this country well in practical every arena. Undercutting this design will, as our national experience has recurrently borne out, weaken our ability to deliver health care in a cost-effective manner rather than strengthen it.

Protect the Present Workforce and Indulge Future Prospects

We have recurrently established that the most essential fiber of a vibrant health care delivery system is its workforce. When it comes to making a career selection, altruism and a concern for others can only take you so far. The medical field is an emotionally tasking and physically draining vocation. The complexity of the material to be mastered is seemingly overwhelming, and the dedication demanded to maintain proficiency is unrelenting. As such, our system *needs* to lure the brightest and most capable minds to this field, because someday, each of our respective lives may depend on the degree of brilliance in the candidates our system fostered. Our system then needs to encourage these highly valuable, resilient and caring people to want to persevere in their endeavors for as long as possible. Our system has precious few commodities with which to achieve these ends: reimbursement, professional independence, growth opportunities, economic stability and minimal administrative drains or distractors. Any system designed to deliver health care must manipulate these factors to maximize recruitment and retention. It is clear that the present proposals for health care reform do neither.

153

The Illegal Immigrant Population

As mentioned previously, the illegal immigrant population poses unique challenges to the health care system in the United States. The strain imparted by approximately 11.8 million unregistered, uninsured and largely poor individuals on our health care system is enormous. The effects of illegal immigration in the United States is far greater in scope, however, than any implications it may have upon the health care system. Issues of national defense, workforce shortages, relations with Mexico, income tax and workers rights are a small sample of the permutations this population carries on our society. Health care policy relating to this population cannot be addressed without formulating a general plan on how the United States wishes to deal with the issue of illegal immigration. Even the countries that are touted as providing universal health care coverage require some sort of legally approved entry process that includes the execution of appropriate registration procedures for someone to benefit from its health care system. For now, the United States has not enacted any such validation process for individuals living in this country illegally.

We should also acknowledge that the establishment of health care coverage is a valuable commodity for individuals living outside of the United States and will serve as further incentive for individuals to enter this country illegally.

It is also clear that the majority of Americans do not favor funding health care services for unauthorized inhabitants. Consequently, as long as the question of government policy towards this population remains unaddressed, any attempt at solving its health care needs will be less than effective.

Julio Gonzalez, M.D.

Keep the Handle of Health Care Costs
Squarely in the Hands of the Consumer

We have previously noted that health care costs have spun to levels of unacceptability. The proponents of health care reform are convinced that through government intervention and greater regulation on quality indicators and expense pattern reviews, it will be able to nickel and dime its way to regaining control of health care expenditure. However, it is more likely that all this approach will accomplish is to create a government bureaucracy that will dwarf Medicare in size.

Although we were unable to identify an expense category that explains the American health care spending spree, we did identify the root cause, consumers spending health care dollars in a highly capitalist system without being held accountable for the size of the account, a concept known as "price insensitivity". True health care reform in this situation is one that places the consumer in charge of determining the price of the product he is going to pay and somehow makes him or her accountable for that charge. There are many ways we could reform the system in order to accomplish this. One is through an increasing reliance on health savings accounts where the consumer is essentially the insurer. Another is to increase the out-of-pocket expenses inherent to a plan, or at least make it a tiered system that decreases the patient's responsibility as the magnitude of the condition increases. Another product could be a combined retirement and health savings account that pays back after a certain age, but carries deductions from the return based on the amount of money the patient uses on health care throughout his life. If cutting corners on expenses for routine medical checkups is a problem, then exceptions to the return reduction scheme can be devised as can rewards for participation in a program of ongoing routine care.

In support of this, health care provider prices should be placed out in the open. This includes allowing physicians the freedom to know the prices being charged by other physicians, a practice that is presently prohibited by federal law. This is the only way that health care providers can compete in a free market system. Insurance companies should not be allowed to set the prices on health care services. This may sound intimidating to insurers, but if the consumer is given a stake on how much he pays and the total amount he is willing to invest in the treatment and evaluation of his condition, third party payers will likely find the price per encounter to not be excessively different from what they are paying now, plus there may be a drop in the total cost of health care consumption.

I am sure that there are countless other strategies insurance and health policy experts can propose with the aim of placing a greater stake of the cost of health care on the consumer while still allowing for access to more involved interventions. These are the ideas regarding health care funding that we should be considering because only by sensitizing the consumer to the price of his purchases, will we stand a chance at regaining control of overall spending.

Level the Playing Field Between Employer-Based and Individual Insurance Plans

Every effort should be made at removing tax incentives that favors an employer-based plan over an individual one. America's reliance on the employer to provide health care coverage is outdated, restrictive to the individual and increasingly less effective at capturing the largest segments of our workforce. Additionally, increasing the fiscal burden on the employer will actually have negative effects on the economy, unemployment levels and mean wages earned. Employer-based insurance plans were never intended to provide massive health care coverage for the population. If we had thought and planned of a way to provide health care coverage to the largest segment of the population, the employer-based system as we know it would likely not be the method selected. There is therefore no reason why we should be keeping it over more effective methods.

Julio Gonzalez, M.D.

Retroactive Reimbursement for Unfunded Care

One of the most financially devastating situations that I come across is the sudden development of disease or injury in an uninsured patient that renders the previously healthy individual unable to work. People who find themselves in this situation are usually young, vibrant individuals who are working for a living, short on money and heavy on good health. In their quest to cut expenses, they decide to forego the expense of medical insurance. Alternatively, they may be working for small businesses which do not fund their insurance for them. When the unthinkable happens, these individuals are unable to afford their medical bills and are unable to work. The result of this situation is predictably disastrous.

One solution we could design that does not universalize medicine is to create a public assistance fund. Through this program, any injured or acutely ill individual becomes eligible for immediate health care benefits in support of the evaluation and treatment of a major condition that elicits costs greater than the patient can afford. The public fund assumes responsibility for payment of these medical bills and affords the patient access to appropriate rehabilitative services. Once the patient is able to return to work, he is then responsible for payment of all medical charges incurred at a pace that is adjusted for his income, but under no circumstances will be zero. This payback effort can be administered by the IRS, who has the ultimate handle on that individual's yearly earnings and his ability to pay. The plan will work retroactively so that the health care providers are reimbursed for their efforts and no longer burdened with the load of paying for the uninsured's health care.

This "individual bailout plan" has a number of advantages. First, it keeps the responsibility for the costs of the health care rendered in the hands of the individual. Secondly, it does not provide "free" insurance. Thirdly, it shifts the burden of funding uninsured patient care away from the provider. Fourth, it helps a person during a time of desperate need, and forces him to pay the investment back once his health is restored.

Insurance Responsibilities

The changes noted in the prior three sections would form the cornerstone for health care coverage reform. Insurance companies would have to redirect their efforts at providing products that fit within the new health care model. However, there are some other provisions that should be included in the health care coverage scheme. There should be no premium adjustments for illnesses that develop without influence from factors outside of the patient's control. Since patients have no control over their age and gender, there should be no age or gender-adjusted influences on premiums. Through price averaging, insurers should be able to arrive at a figure that will cover their expenses without relying on such adjustments. Gone is the uninsurable patient. However, insurance should offer discounts or rewards to enrollees who are engaged in treatment and life-style interventions that lower their risks for certain illnesses. Additionally, there should be no waiting period for coverage on preexisting conditions. Instead, there should be minimum lengths of contract agreements for patients with preexisting conditions .

Some of these restrictions on premium policy requirements may sound intimidating to insurers. However, there are two answers to their objections.

The first is that the insurance company is in business to facilitate health care access to the individual. There is no qualifier on individual, such as healthy, female, or young. If that's what they are in business to do then they need to provide the service and take the good risk with the bad. Secondly, be aware that these are restrictions placed in a milieu of a larger scheme that makes the patient/consumer a co-stakeholder with the insurance company. This co-responsibility will serve as a powerful check on the overall price of the coverage insurers deliver. The general market environment will ensure that health care remains an acceptable risk for the insurer.

Get Rid of the SGR

The SGR as a formula for provider reimbursement is so flawed it should be abandoned. Either a new plan allowing the consumer to select the rate it desires from competing providers should be implemented or another formula must be devised that will account for the true inflationary trends dealing with the costs of delivering care. As noted previously, with the present scheme, every time the flawed SGR is corrected by Congressional action, the government spends itself increasingly into debt. As the process continues, there will come a day when Congress will stop overriding these calculated cuts in physician reimbursement and a massive exodus of physicians from the Medicare system will ensue. We are much better off correcting the formula than continuing to live with its consequences.

Prevent Preventive Medicine Efforts From Playing A Role in Cost-Containment

It's a sexy health policy phrase conjuring up images of fit joggers running through some scenic trail while drinking mineral spring water and eating nutrition bars, and it makes the promoter of such programs appear to be really concerned for the wellbeing of others and really intelligent about how to do this. However, the fact is that preventive medicine is expensive and many of the interventions devised may not be saving much money at all. There are some interventions that truly do prevent the appearance of disease, but these are not the attractive, popular ones that one might envision. Truly effective preventive medicine in an organized scale is limited to pap-smear screens, smoking cessation efforts, obesity-prevention education, work-environment modifications and periodic physical examinations with targeted interventions such as colonoscopies, DEXA scans, mammograms and so forth. Even when successful, all these efforts accomplish is to shift the expense of health care to another disease appearing later in time. Although preventive medicine is an invaluable tool for the public health expert and the individual, it plays a very small role for the economist and should not play a major role in the effort towards cutting health care costs.

Julio Gonzalez, M.D.

Medical Malpractice

There is a large amount of room for improvement in the medical malpractice arena. Enacting changes that will protect the physician from unsubstantiated lawsuits will go a long way towards diminishing the costs of health care and allow for the development of progressive innovations in how health care issues are addressed. Some states have met with success in curtailing the hostile litigation environment by enacting limits on the amount juries can allocate on non-expense grounds such as pain and suffering. These legislations are to be encouraged. Additionally, there should be checks instituted that stop unsubstantiated actions from proceeding. One of these is to require that cases be reviewed for merit by a board of health care providers whose majority is comprised of clinicians. By providing this funnel, the likelihood that unsubstantiated cases actually make it to court will be further diminished. It will also serve to decrease the amount of money and time a physician spends defending meritless cases. Another reform is the establishment of health courts specific to the practice of medicine. These are courts that review medical cases and whose juries are composed of health care providers well-versed in the field of medicine. The judges of these health courts also undergo enhanced training in medical issues. In order to help guarantee the fairness of the court, the opinions of the health care experts seated in the jury should be reviewable by their respective professional societies or boards for potential ethics violations. Any ethical breaches would then be severely punished and nullify the outcome of the case. Additionally, plaintiffs who sue over medical cases should be accountable for court costs, cost of defense and lost income for the defendant should a defense verdict be reached. This will help ensure the plaintiffs confidence in his contention prior to proceeding with civil action. Finally, in the new practice environment physicians should not be held liable for unfavorable outcomes that arise from decisions made by patients based on expense of services considerations, provided that the physician supply the patient with written information about the potential consequences of the patient's decision. This measure frees the physician from liability incurred from practicing in a cost-containment environment.

Julio Gonzalez, M.D.

Cut the Public Health Funding to Futile Cases

We have already established that exorbitant amounts of money are paid every year in interventions afforded to patients in their last year of life. Research should be undertaken towards the creation of a health index that predicts the likelihood of limited longevity. Once the patient reaches that health index score, government and insurance funding designed to cure major illnesses such as cancer should be discontinued. For the sake of the patient, his loved ones and our economy, efforts should be redirected from curative to supportive. The decision over spending money for that care is removed from the provider and patient alike. After all, it is the third-party payer's money, and the payer should therefore be free to withhold funding for curative care in cases that are obviously futile to pursue. Of course, the cutoff score on such an index should be sufficiently high to satisfy reasonable ethical concerns, but not so high as to disarm the program completely. It is important to note that although this index should be influenced by the age of the patient, chronological age should not be the sole determinant of the final score.

For example, an otherwise active 90 year old who

still lives independently, drives a car, shops for her own food and has a heart attack should be scoring sufficiently low on the health index to qualify her to be treated for her heart attack.

On the other hand an independent-living 85 year old patient on Coumadin for atrial fibrillation with a history of a heart attack, coronary artery and congestive heart failure who develops a sarcoma that is potentially curable with a combination of aggressive surgical intervention, chemotherapy and radiation should not have those services covered by public or private health insurance funds. Such an intervention is futile and even if successful will only serve to add a few painful months to this patient's life. The patient can still fund this intervention out of his own pocket, although admittedly the exorbitant expense of his treatment would likely be so high as to make such an alternative prohibitive. However, in this case the public funding system, whether from government of private sources, should be free to acknowledge the reality of our mortality and accept that pursuing expensive, curative interventions is no longer of value to society or to the patient. Instead, this patient and his family should be assisted in procuring supportive and comfort measures which will be covered by the appropriate third-party payer.

CHAPTER 11:

SO WHAT'S THE TRUTH ABOUT THE PRESENT PLANS FOR HEALTH CARE REFORM?

The truth about the present plan to reform health care is that it is a concerted effort by individuals bent on radically changing the way health care is delivered in this country. It is a reform that fails to acknowledge the incredible accomplishments of our health care system and focuses instead on its shortcomings, all with the goal of increasing the government's power and influence over its citizenry.

The truth about the present health care reform scheme is that it considers only one approach to addressing the shortcomings of our health care system even with the warnings afforded to it by historical record and the experiences of other countries. It is an approach that has been undertaken with minimal stakeholder participation and one that will damage morale within the health care workforce leading many to consider early retirement. It is a health care reform plan that discourages the brightest minds of the newer generations from filling in the gaps created by the attrition it will inevitably cause.

The truth about health care reform is that it radically overhauls a system in order to address specific concerns within it, akin to using a cannonball to kill a fly. It is a reform plan that relies on flawed assumptions and misinterpretation of fact and data in order to defend its ideals. It is a plan that purposely confuses health care deficiencies with deficiencies of life style and poverty, and aims to take over those lifestyles in an exuberant government power grab disguised as a caring and altruistic venture.

If the truth be told, it is a proposal that one could argue does not constitute reform at all, but merely an emulation and reproduction of the Canadian and European health care systems that are wrestling with issues of unresponsiveness, rationing of care and an inability to create physicians from candidates recruited within their borders.

The truth about health care reform is that it is almost guaranteed to create a system of greater administrative burden, greater cost, and greater government intrusion into the daily affairs of the American citizen. It is a system that distrusts every instinct that served to drive this country into becoming the leading socioeconomic entity the world has ever known, as if somehow those forces of freedom to succeed, freedom to fail and freedom to profit were wrong and unjust. It is a reform plan that must be resisted, but not just with blaring criticisms and truthful analyses, but through the thoughtful consideration of alternative ideas that promote reliance upon human motivation and individual accountability. These principles will work for health care, just like they worked in building a nation.

REFERENCES

1.   U.S. Census Bureau, "Income, Poverty, and Health Insurance Coverage in the United States: 2007" U.S. Census Bureau, Pp 19-20. http://www.census.gov/prod/2008pubs/p60-235.pdf.

2.   U.S. Census Bureau, "Income, Poverty, and Health Insurance Coverage in the United States: 2007" U.S. Census Bureau, Pg 20. http://www.census.gov/prod/2008pubs/p60-235.pdf.

3.   U.S. Census Bureau, "Income, Poverty, and Health Insurance Coverage in the United States: 2007" U.S. Census Bureau, Table 6. http://www.census.gov/prod/2008pubs/p60-235.pdf.

4.   US Department of Health and Services. Bureau of Health Professions. "Physician Supply and Demand: Projections to 2020". October, 2006. ftp://ftp.hrsa.gov/bhpr/workforce/PhysicianForecastingPaperfinal.pdf

5.   US Department of Health and Services. Bureau of Health Professions. "National Center for Work Force Analysis: US Health Workforce Factbook". Table 201. http://bhpr.hrsa.gov/healthworkforce/reports/factbook02/FB102.htm

6.   Association of American Medical Colleges. Table 1. http://services.aamc.org/tsfreports/report_median.cfm?year_of_study=2009

7.   College Board. "College Prices 2008-2009" http://www.collegeboard.com/student/pay/add-it-up/4494.html

8.   Association of American Colleges. "Recent Studies and Reports on Physician Shortages in the US." October, 2008. http://www.aamc.org/workforce/recentworkforcestudies2008.pdf

9.   Brooks, R.G.; Menachemi, N.: Florida's Physician Workforce: Preliminary Results From a Statewide Survey." October, 2007.

10.   Association of American Colleges. "Table 4: Matriculants to US Schools by State of Legal Residence 1997-2008." http://www.aamc.org/data/facts/2008/2008slrmat.htm

11.   Aki, E.A.; Mustafa, R.; Bdair, F.; Shunemann H: "The United State Physician Workforce and International Medical Graduates: Trends and Characteristics." Journ. Gen. Int. Med. Vol 22. No. 2. February 22, 2007. Pp 264-268

12.   Hart, G. L.; Skillman, S. M.; Fordyce, M.; Thompson, M.; Hagopian, A.; Konrad. T. R.: "Physicians in the United States: Changes Since 1981."

Health Affairs. Vol. 26. No. 4. April, 2007. Pp. 1159-1169.

13.   Morris, A. L.; Phillips, R. L.; Fryer Jr., G. E.; Green, L. A.; Mullan, F.: "International Medica Graduates in the United States of America: An Exploration of Professional Characteristics and Attitudes." Human Resources for Health. Vol. 4:17. July, 26, 2006. http://www.human-resources-health. com/content/pdf/1478-4491-4-18.pdf

14.   World Health Organization. The World Health Organization Report 2000. Health Systems: Improving Performance. World Health Organization. Geneva, Switzerland. Table 6. http://www.who.int/whr/2000/en/whr00_ en.pdf.

15.   Kenen, J.: "Health Reform: Supply and Demand Adds Up to Crisis in the ER." New American Foundation. August 17, 2008. http://www. newamerica.net/blog/topics/emergency-rooms?page=1.

16.   Australian Institute for Health and Welfare. "6 International Developments in Health Sector Performance Analysis." Australian Institute for Health and Welfare. 2003 Figure 6.2. http://www.aihw.gov.au/publications/ hwi/nrhspi03/nrhspi03-c11.pdf.

17.   Blendon, R. J.; Kim, M.; Benson, J. M.: "The Public Versus the World Health Organization On Health System Performance. Health Affairs. Vol 20. No. 3. May/June, 2001. Pp. 10-20. Exhibit 2. http://content. healthaffairs.org/cgi/content/full/20/3/10.

18.   Hoeffer, M; Rytina, N; Baker, B.C.: "Estimates of the Unauthorized Population Residing in the United States: January 2007," Department of Homeland Security September, 2008. Pg. 1. http://www.dhs.gov/xlibrary/ assets/statistics/publications/ois_ill_pe_2007.pdf

19.   Time magazine: "Time Magazine/SRBI March 29-30, 2006." Time Magazine Q #8. http://www.srbi.com/TimePoll_Final_Report-2006-03-31.pdf

20.   The Kaiser Commission. "The Uninsured. A Primer. Key Facts About Americans Without Insurance" October, 2008. http://www.kff.org/ uninsured/upload/7451-04.pdf

21.   Health Insurance Resource Center. "Risk Pools for the Medically-Uninsurable." http://www.healthinsurance.org/risk_pools/

22.   Annual Estimates of the Population for the United States, Regions, States, and Puerto Rico: April 1, 2000 to July 1, 2007 (NST-EST2007-01). http://www.census.gov/popest/states/NST-ann-est.html

23.   Truman, HS. "Presidential Address to Congress of November 19, 1945. http://www.cms.hhs.gov/History/Downloads/CMSPresidentsSpeeches.pdf

24.   Centers for Medicare and Medicaid Services. "Key Milestones in CMS Programs. Centers for Medicare and Medicaid Services. http://www.cms.hhs.gov/History/Downloads/CMSProgramKeyMilestones.pdf

25.   U.S. Census Bureau, "Income, Poverty, and Health Insurance Coverage in the United States: 2007" U.S. Census Bureau, Pg 22. http://www.census.gov/prod/2008pubs/p60-235.pdf.

26.   Jones, S. B.: "Medicare Influence on Private Insurance: Good or Ill?" Health Care Financing Rev. Vol. 18. No. 2. 1996 Pp 153-161. http://ssa.gov/history/pdf/MedicareInfluencePrivateInsurance.pdf

27.   Murphy, D. S.: From Barefoot Boy to Doc...My Journey. Morningside Press. Venice, Florida. 2002. Pg. 159.

28.   Finkelstein, Amy. "The Aggregate Effects of Health Insurance: Evidence from the Introduction of Medicare." National Bureau of Economic Research. NBER Working Paper No. 11619. September, 2005.

29.   Nesvisky, M.: "Medicare and its Impact." National Bureau of Economic Impact. http://www.nber.org/digest/apr06/w11609.html.

30.   Centers for Medicare and Medicaid Services. "Estimated Sustainable Growth Rate and Conversion Factor, for Medicare Payments to Physicians 2009." Sustainable Growth Rates and Conversion Factors. Overview. Centers for Medicare and Medicaid Services. http://www.cms.hhs.gov/SustainableGRatesConFact/Downloads/sgr2009f.pdf
31.   Perlin, J. B.; Kolodner, R. M.; Roswell, R. H.: "The Veterans Administration: Quality, Value, Accountability, and Information as Transforming Strategies for Patient-Centered Care." Am. J. Managed Care. Vol. 10. No. 11. Pg. 828-836.

32.   Congressional Budget Office: "Limiting Tort Liability for Medical Malpractice." Congressional Budget Office. January 8, 2004. Pg. 1. http://www.cbo.gov/ftpdocs/49xx/doc4968/01-08-MedicalMalpractice.pdf

33.   Congressional Budget Office: "Limiting Tort Liability for Medical Malpractice." Congressional Budget Office. January 8, 2004. Pg. 4. http://www.cbo.gov/ftpdocs/49xx/doc4968/01-08-MedicalMalpractice.pdf

34.   Congressional Budget Office: "Limiting Tort Liability for Medical Malpractice." Congressional Budget Office. January 8, 2004. Pg. 6. http://www.cbo.gov/ftpdocs/49xx/doc4968/01-08-MedicalMalpractice.pdf

35.   Baucus, M: "Call to Action-Health Reform 2009" Senate Finance Committee Chairman; November 12, 2008. Pp. 74-75. http://finance.senate.gov/healthreform2009/finalwhitepaper.pdf

36.   Blumenthal, P.: "More Doctors in Texas After Malpractice Caps." The New York Times. October 5, 2007. http://www.nytimes.com/2007/10/05/us/05doctors.html?_r=1

37.   Baucus, M: "Call to Action-Health Reform 2009" Senate Finance Committee Chairman; November 12, 2008. Pg. 13. http://finance.senate.gov/healthreform2009/finalwhitepaper.pdf

38.   Baucus, M: "Call to Action-Health Reform 2009" Senate Finance Committee Chairman; November 12, 2008. Pg. 2. http://finance.senate.gov/healthreform2009/finalwhitepaper.pdf

39.   Baucus, M: "Call to Action-Health Reform 2009" Senate Finance Committee Chairman; November 12, 2008. Pg. 17. http://finance.senate.gov/healthreform2009/finalwhitepaper.pdf

40.   Baucus, M: "Call to Action-Health Reform 2009" Senate Finance Committee Chairman; November 12, 2008. Pg. 30. http://finance.senate.gov/healthreform2009/finalwhitepaper.pdf

41.   Baucus, M: "Call to Action-Health Reform 2009" Senate Finance Committee Chairman; November 12, 2008. Pg. 65. http://finance.senate.gov/healthreform2009/finalwhitepaper.pdf

42.   Time magazine: "Time Magazine/SRBI Jan 24-6, 2006." Time Magazine Q #26 http://www.srbi.com/TimePoll3738-Final%20Report-2006-01-27--8.05am.pdf

43.   CIA The World Factbook. https://www.cia.gov/library/publications/the-world-factbook/appendix/appendix-b.html

44.   World Health Organization. The World Health Organization Report 2000. Health Systems: Improving Performance. World Health Organization. Geneva, Switzerland. Annex Table 1. http://www.who.int/whr/2000/en/whr00_en.pdf.

45.   Baucus, M: "Call to Action-Health Reform 2009" Senate Finance Committee Chairman; November 12, 2008. P. 31. http://finance.senate.gov/healthreform2009/finalwhitepaper.pdf

46.   WHO Statistical Information System (WHOSIS). http://www.who.int/whosis/indicators/compendium/2008/3mr5/en/

47.   Center for Medicine in the Public Interest. "Infant Mortality and Premature Birth." BigGovHealth. Center for Medicine in the Public Interest. http://www.biggovhealth.org/resource/myths-facts/infant-mortality-and-premature-birth/

48.   Centers for Disease Control: "Increasing Infant Mortality Among Very Low Birthweight Infants, Delaware 1994 Through 2000." Morbidity and Mortality Weekly Report. Vol 52(36) September 12, 2003. Pp. 862-863. http://www.cdc.gov/mmwr/preview/mmwrhtml/mm5236a3.htm

49.   MacDorman, M. F.; Matthews, T. J.: "Recent Trends in Infant Mortality in the United States." National Center for Health Statistics. Centers for Disease Control. Number 9. October, 2008. http://www.cdc.gov/nchs/data/databriefs/db09.htm

50.   Gould, E.; Smeeding, T.; Wolfe, B.: "Trends in the Health of the Poor and the Near Poor: Have the Poor and Near Poor Been Catching Up to the Non Poor in the Last 25 Years?" Paper Presented Annual Meeting of the Economics of Population Healtt: Inaugural Conference American Society of Health Economists. Madison WI June 4, 2006. http://www.allacademic.com/meta/p_mla_apa_research_citation/0/9/3/4/4/p93442_index.html.

51.   Samartin, C.; Ng, E.: Blackwell, D.; Gentleman, J.; Martinez, M.; Simile, M.: "Joint Canada/United states Survey of Health, 2002=2003". Statistics Canada. Centers for Disease Control. 2003. http://www.cdc.gov/nchs/data/nhis/jcush_analyticalreport.pdf.

52.   Centers for Medicare and Medicaid Services. "National Health Expenditure Data." Centers for Medicare and Medicaid Services. http://www.cms.hhs.gov/NationalHealthExpendData/01_Overview.asp#TopOfPage.

53.   American Medical Association. "Administrative Costs of Health Care Coverage." Series on the AMA Proposal for Reform. Pg 1. http://www.ama-assn.org/ama1/pub/upload/mm/478/admincosts.pdf

54.   American Medical Association. "Administrative Costs of Health Care Coverage." Series on the AMA Proposal for Reform. Pg 2. http://www.ama-assn.org/ama1/pub/upload/mm/478/admincosts.pdf

55.   Litow, M.; The Technical Committee for The Council for Affordable Health Insurance: "Rhetoric vs. Reality: Comparing Public and Private Health Care Administrative Costs." The Council for Affordable Health Insurance. March, 2004. http://heartland.temp.siteexecutive.com/pdf/32923a.pdf.

56.   Matthews, M.: "Medicare's Hidden Administrative Costs: A Comparison of Medicare and the Private Sector." Council for Affordable Health Insurance. January 10, 2006. Pg. 1. http://www.cahi.org/cahi_contents/resources/pdf/CAHI_Medicare_Admin_Final_Publication.pdf.

57.   Matthews, M.: "Medicare's Hidden Administrative Costs: A Comparison of Medicare and the Private Sector." Council for Affordable Health Insurance. January 10, 2006. Pg. 11. http://www.cahi.org/cahi_contents/resources/pdf/CAHI_Medicare_Admin_Final_Publication.pdf.

58.   United States Senate website. Membership roster for the Senate Finance Committee December 2, 2008. http://finance.senate.gov/sitepages/committee.htm

59.   Baucus, M: "Reforming America's Health Care System: A Call to Action" Senate Finance Committee Chairman; November 12, 2008. http://finance.senate.gov/healthreform2009/finalwhitepaper.pdf

60.   "High Health Care Costs: A States Perspective." United States Senate Finance Committee Hearing. held on October 21, 2008. http://finance.senate.gov/sitepages/hearing102108.htm

61.   "Covering the Uninsured: Making Health Insurance Markets Work." United States Senate Finance Committee Hearing. Held on September 23, 2008. http://finance.senate.gov/sitepages/hearing092308.htm

62.   "Aligning Incentives: The Case for Delivery System Reform." United States Senate Finance Committee Hearing. Held on September 16, 2008. http://finance.senate.gov/sitepages/hearing091608.htm

63.   "Improving Health Care Quality: An Integral Step Toward Health Reform." United States Senate Finance Committee Hearing. Held on September 9, 2008. http://finance.senate.gov/sitepages/hearing090908.htm

64.   "Health Benefits in the Tax Code: The Right Incentives." United States Senate Finance Committee Hearing. Held on July 31, 2008. http://finance.senate.gov/sitepages/hearing073108.htm

65. "The Right Care at the Right Time: Levering Innovation to Improve Health Care Quality for All Americans." United States Senate Finance Committee Hearing. Held on July 17, 2008. http://finance.senate.gov/sitepages/hearing071708.htm

66. "47 Million and Counting: Why the Health Care Marketplace is Broken." United States Senate Finance Committee Hearing. Held on June 10, 2008. http://finance.senate.gov/sitepages/hearing061008.htm

67. "Rising Costs, Low Quality in Health Care: The Necessity for Reform." United States Senate Finance Committee Hearing. Held on June 3, 2008. http://finance.senate.gov/sitepages/hearing060308.htm

68. "Seizing the New Opportunity for Health Reform." United States Senate Finance Committee Hearing. Held on May 6, 2008. http://finance.senate.gov/sitepages/hearing050608.htm
69. "Subcommittee on Health Care Hearing on Covering Uninsured Children: The Impact of the August 17 CHIP Directive." United States Senate Finance Committee Hearing. Held on April 9, 2008. http://finance.senate.gov/sitepages/hearing040908.htm

70. "Selling to Seniors: The Need for Accountability and Oversight of Marketing and Sales by Medicare Private Plans (Part 2)." United States Senate Finance Committee Hearing. Held on February 13, 2008. http://finance.senate.gov/sitepages/hearing021308.htm

71. "Selling to Seniors: The Need for Accountability and Oversight of Marketing and Sales by Medicare Private Plans (Part 1)." United States Senate Finance Committee Hearing. Held on February 7, 2008. http://finance.senate.gov/sitepages/hearing020708.htm

72. "Private Fee for Service Plans in Medicare Advantage: A Closer Look." United States Senate Finance Committee Hearing. Held on January 30, 2008. http://finance.senate.gov/sitepages/hearing013008.htm

73. Personal Communication Mr. David Lovett, J.D. December 2, 2008.

74. United States Senate website. About the Senate Health Education Labor and Pensions Committee December 2, 2008. http://help.senate.gov/About.html

75. MedPAC website. About the MedPAC. Commission Members. December 2, 2008. http://www.medpac.gov/commission.cfm

183

76.   MedPAC Website. About the MedPAC. Commissioners' Biographies Members. December 2, 2008. http://www.medpac.gov/biographies.cfm

77.   Pear, Robert.: "Ending Its Secrecy, White House Lists Health-Care Panel.: New York Times. March 27, 1993. http://query.nytimes.com/gst/fullpage.html?res=9F0CE7DA1131F934A15750C0A965958260&sec=&spon=&pagewanted=3

78.   Baucus, M: "Call to Action-Health Reform 2009" Senate Finance Committee Chairman; November 12, 2008. Pg. 16. http://finance.senate.gov/healthreform2009/finalwhitepaper.pdf

79.   Pauly, M; Percy, A; Herring, B.: "Individual Vs. Job-Based Health Insurance: Weighing the Pros and Cons." Health Affairs. Vol 18. No. 6. Pp. 28-44. http://content.healthaffairs.org/cgi/reprint/18/6/28.pdf

80.   The Hamilton Project. "Evolving Beyond Traditional Employer-Sponsored Health Insurance." Policy Brief No. 2007-06. May, 2007 Pg. 2. http://www.brookings.edu/papers/2007/~/media/Files/rc/papers/2007/05healthcare_butler/200705butler_pb.pdf

81.   Butler, S. M:. "Evolving Beyond Traditional Employer-Sponsored Health Insurance." Discussion Paper. The Brookings Institution. No. 2007-06. May, 2007 Pg. 2. http://www3.brookings.edu/es/hamilton/200705butler.pdf

82.   Klein, S.: "Quality Matters: Pay for Performance in Medicare." The Commonwealth Fund. September 21, 2006. Vol 20. http://www.commonwealthfund.org/publications/publications_show.htm?doc_id=402822

83.   Nidiry, M. A. J.; Gozu, A.; Carrese, J. A..; Wright, S. M.: "The Closure of a Medical Practice Forces Older Patients to Make Difficult Decisions: A Qualitative Study of a Natural Experiment. Journal of General Internal Medicine. Vol. 23. No. 10. October, 2008. Pp1576-1580. http://www.springerlink.com/content/2431340673332330/

84.   Health Care Renewal. "On Disparities of Primary Care and Proceduralist Physicians. Health Care renewal. March 13, 2007. http://hcrenewal.blogspot.com/2007/03/on-disparities-between-reimbursement-of.html

85.   Hamilton, D. P.: "Overtreatment in Action: $30 Billion Wasted on Unnecessary MRI, CT Scans." BNET Health care. BNET Industries. August 29, 2008. http://industry.bnet.com/health care/1000138/overtreatment-in-action-30-billion-wasted-on-unnecessary-mri-ct-scans/.

86.   Boschert, S.: "MRI Overused in Assessing Knee Osteoarthritis." Internal Medicine News. May 1, 2008. http://www.articlearchives.com/ health-care/medical-allied-health-specialties-orthopedics/186062-1.html

87.   Jauhar, S.: "The Pitfalls of Linking Doctors' Pay to Performance." The New York Times. September 8, 2008. http://www.nytimes. com/2008/09/09/health/09essa.html?_r=1&scp=1&sq=Dr.%20Sandeep%20 Jauhar%20pay%20for%20performance&st=cse

88.   Cunningnham, P. J.; May, J. H.: "Medicaid Patients Increasingly Concentrated Amongst Physicians. Tracking Report Number 16." Center for Studying Health System Change. August, 2006. http://www.hschange.com/ CONTENT/866/.

89.   Freking, K.: "Doctors Taking Less Medicaid Patients." The Washington Post. August 17, 2006. http://www.washingtonpost.com/wp-dyn/ content/article/2006/08/17/AR2006081700088.html.

90.   KeyeTV.com. "ER: In Critical Condition: Medicaid Patients in the ER." Keye TV. October 29, 2007. http://www.keyetv.com/news/local/story. aspx?content_id=DD4620F6-0CA8-475B-9BEC-96A56AD78299&gsa=true.

91.   American Medical Association. "Member Connect Survey: Physicians' Reaction to the Medicare Physicians Payment Cuts." American Medical Association April/May, 2007. http://vocuspr.vocus.com/VocusPR30/ ViewAttachment.aspx?EID=rhvBPIv6TFrQEnOBF28gCjf4F99FXMmV9yIvt y90Xmc%3d.

92.   Florida Department of Health. "2008 Florida Physician Workforce Annual Report. In Response to the Provisions of Section 381.4018, Florida Statutes." Florida Department of Health. November 1, 2008.. http://doh.state. fl.us/rw_Bulletins/WorkforceRept08.pdf

93.   Florida Department of Health. "2008 Florida Physician Workforce Annual Report. In Response to the Provisions of Section 381.4018, Florida Statutes." Florida Department of Health. November 1, 2008. Figure 10. Pg 5. http://doh.state.fl.us/rw_Bulletins/WorkforceRept08.pdf

94.   Florida Department of Health. "2008 Florida Physician Workforce Annual Report. In Response to the Provisions of Section 381.4018, Florida Statutes." Florida Department of Health. November 1, 2008. Figure 10. Pg 10. http://doh.state.fl.us/rw_Bulletins/WorkforceRept08.pdf

95.   Garcia-Perez, M. A.; Amaya, C.; Otero, A.: "Physicians' Migration in Europe: An Overview of the Current Situation." BMC Health Serv. Res. Vol. 7. 2007. http://www.pubmedcentral.nih.gov/articlerender.fcgi?artid=2248190.

96.   McKinsey Global Institute. Accounting for the Cost of US Health Care: A New Look at Why American Spend More." McKinsey & Company. December, 2008. Pg.10. http://www.mckinsey.com/mgi/reports/pdfs/health care/US_healthcare_report.pdf.

97.   Reinhardt, U.: "Why Does U.S. Health Care Cost So Much? (Part III: Ah Aging Population Isn't the Reason). Economix. December 5, 2008. http://economix.blogs.nytimes.com/2008/12/05/why-does-us-health-care-cost-so-much-part-iii-an-aging-population-isnt-the-reason/

98.   Reinhardt, U.: "Doctors' Salaries and the Cost of Health Care.. Economix. November 14, 2008. Reinhardt, U.: "Why Does U.S. Health Care Cost So Much? (Part III: Ah Aging Population Isn't the Reason). Economix. December 5, 2008. http://economix.blogs.nytimes.com/2008/12/05/why-does-us-health-care-cost-so-much-part-iii-an-aging-population-isnt-the-reason/

99.   McKinsey Global Institute. Accounting for the Cost of US Health Care: A New Look at Why American Spend More." McKinsey & Company. December, 2008. Pg.11. http://www.mckinsey.com/mgi/reports/pdfs/health care/US_healthcare_report.pdf.

100.   Centers for Medicare and Medicaid Services. "Historical NHE, Including Sponsor Analysis, 2006:" National Health Expenditure Data. Centers for Medicare and Medicaid Services. Page last modified December 23, 2008. http://www.cms.hhs.gov/NationalHealthExpendData/25_NHE_Fact_Sheet.asp#TopOfPage

101.   Baucus, M: "Call to Action-Health Reform 2009" Senate Finance Committee Chairman; November 12, 2008. Pg. 31. http://finance.senate.gov/healthreform2009/finalwhitepaper.pdf

102.   Woods, D.: "The Chimera of Preventive Medicine in Reducing Health Care Costs." The Canadian Medical Association Journal. Vol 129. November 1, 1983. http://www.pubmedcentral.nih.gov/picrender.fcgi?artid=1875861&blobtype=pdf.

103.   Cohen, J. T.; Neumann, P. J.; Weinstein, M.C.: "Does Preventive Medicine Save Money? Health Economics and the Presidential Candidates." New England Journal of Medicine. February 14, 2008. Vol. 358. No. 7. Pp. 661-3. Woods, D.: "The Chimera of Preventive Medicine in Reducing Health Care Costs." The Canadian Medical Association Journal. Vol 129. November

1, 1983. http://www.pubmedcentral.nih.gov/picrender.fcgi?artid=1875861&bl
obtype=pdf.

104.   Appleby, J.: "Debate Surrounds End-of-Life Health Care Costs.:
USA Today October 19, 2008. http://www.usatoday.com/money/industries/
health/2006-10-18-end-of-life-costs_x.htm.

105.   Centers for Medicare and Medicaid Services. "Estimated Sustainable
Growth Rate and Conversion Factor, for Medicare Payments to Physicians
2009." Sustainable Growth Rates and Conversion Factors. Overview.
Centers for Medicare and Medicaid Services. http://www.cms.hhs.gov/
SustainableGRatesConFact/Downloads/sgr2009f.pdf.

Also by Julio Gonzalez, M.D.

Dictionary of Orthopaedic Terminology

(with Saul Bernstein, M.D. and Deborah Collins)

Journal of Orthopaedic History